# SYNOPSIS OF NEUROLOGY

# SYNOPSIS OF NEUROLOGY

RICHARD LECHTENBERG, MD
Acting Chairman
Department of Neurology
The Long Island College Hospital

Associate Professor of Clinical Neurology
State University of New York
Health Science Center at Brooklyn

Brooklyn, New York

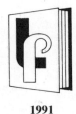

Lea & Febiger

1991

Indiana University
Library
Northwest

Philadelphia  •  London

Lea & Febiger
200 Chester Field Parkway
Malvern, Pennsylvania 19355
U.S.A.
(215) 251-2230
1-800-444-1785

Lea & Febiger (UK) Ltd.
145a Croydon Road
Beckenham, Kent BR3 3RB
U.K.

**Cover:**
Angiogram of intracranial vessels performed to locate the tip of a knife that entered through the left orbit. The unfortunate woman on whom this study was obtained was stabbed repeatedly during a dispute with her husband. She arrived at the emergency room with 4 knives still embedded in her head and neck. Despite the position of the knife seen on this roentgenogram, this woman had no loss of vision or significant intracranial bleeding.

**Library of Congress Cataloging-in-Publication Data**

Lechtenberg, Richard.
  Synopsis of neurology/Richard Lechtenberg.
    p.  cm.
  Includes index.
  ISBN 0-8121-1356-X
  1. Neurology—Handbooks, manuals, etc. 2. Nervous system—
Diseases—Handbooks, manuals, etc.  I. Title.
  [DNLM: 1. Nervous System Diseases.  WL 100 L459s]
RC355.L43  1991
616.8—dc20
DNLM/DLC
for Library of Congress                                          90-6387
                                                             CIP

Reprints of chapters may be purchased from Lea & Febiger in quantities of 100 or more.

Printed in the United States of America
Print Number: 5    4    3    2    1

*To*
*Dr. Lewis P. Rowland*

# Preface

The *Synopsis of Neurology* is a distillation of facts, theories, observations, and impressions that currently are important or useful in neurologic practice. It is organized primarily around signs and symptoms, because that is what the physician must deal with when he or she first sees the patient. A few topics, such as vascular disease, neoplasms, and congenital disorders, are treated separately because most physicians observing a weak leg or a large head want to know more than that they are faced with a stroke or hydrocephalus. Individuals with medical school training, but without sophistication in neurology, will find this synopsis useful as a guide to approaching and managing common neurologic problems. This book is intended to help the house officer reacquaint himself or herself with diagnostic approaches and therapeutic regimens for a variety of neurologic problems and to familiarize the medical student with neurologic syndromes and sequelae.

The drug recommendations listed in the tables reflect the current consensus among neurologists. In some areas no consensus exists, in which cases the most probable answers are provided.

Today's facts rapidly become yesterday's misconceptions in all areas of medicine, and determining which facts are most likely to endure is as difficult in neurology as in any other specialty. To present only the most established ideas would be cowardly and tedious. Consequently, this book tries to provide a glimpse of where thinking in several areas is going, as well as where that thinking is currently.

*Brooklyn, New York*                                      Richard Lechtenberg

# Contents

# Chapter 1
# Examining Patients

The neurologic examination starts with observation of the patient's appearance and activity. Abnormalities of affect, language, movements, strength, and other neurologic characteristics are usually apparent on first meeting the patient. Facial asymmetry, gait problems, comprehension problems, tremors, nystagmus, and clumsiness may be evident even before being specifically sought. Even if no neurologic abnormalities are detected initially, deficits may appear on a more systematic neurologic evaluation.

This neurologic evaluation should assess the patient's mental status, cranial nerve function, motor function, sensation, coordination, and reflexes. If the patient cannot cooperate, either because of age, level of consciousness, or psychiatric problems, the evaluation should focus on neurologic abilities, such as reflexes, eye movements, and involuntary limb movements, which require little or no patient cooperation. The examiner always should check for gross neurologic deficits, such as flaccid weakness of a limb, persistent deviation of the eyes to one side, insensitivity to painful stimuli, or failure to respond to visual threats.

## HISTORY

What the patient recalls about his or her illness should be checked for accuracy and completeness with friends, relatives, or anyone else familiar with the patient. Problems with strength, sensation, hearing, speech, swallowing, vision, balance, coordination, and memory should be asked about specifically. Sexual disorders, bladder or bowel incontinence, and episodes of amnesia are rarely mentioned by the patient unless very direct questions are asked.

Any systemic problems, past operations, and past hospitalizations must be taken into consideration (Table 1-1). Travel, recent immunizations, medications, and dietary practices are all worth knowing. Trips outside the continental United States may have exposed the patient to schistosomiasis, leaving him at risk for leg weakness and numbness from spinal cord damage. A recent immunization may have triggered a Guillain-Barré syndrome of ascending paralysis without sensory impairment. Antihypertensive medication overdose may be responsible for recurrent fainting. Strict vegetarians may develop peripheral nerve dysfunctions if their choices of foods are too limited.

If the patient cannot provide a history, information must be gleaned from ambulance staff, emergency room workers, and other individuals who saw the patient during the evolution of his or her problem. The sequence and speed of the patient's deterioration may help establish the diagnosis and dictate the treatment. While the patient is under medical observation, changes in the neurologic

TABLE 1-1.  *Examining the Patient with a Neurologic Complaint*

| History | Systemic Examination | Neurologic Examination |
|---|---|---|
| Change in consciousness | Heart murmurs or arrhythmias | Level of consciousness |
| Hallucinations or delusions | Hypertension | Cognitive and affective disorders |
| Change in speech | Cutaneous stigmata | Speech or language abnormalities |
| Transient signs or symptoms | Café-au-lait spots | Cranial nerve deficits |
| Focal weakness or numbness | Ash-leaf spots | Gait, strength, and tone |
| Tremors or clumsiness | Telangiectasia | Sensory function |
| Underlying conditions | Port-wine spots | Coordination |
| Travel history | Metabolic abnormalities | Tremors or dysmetria |
| Hospitalizations | Hyperglycemia | Tendon reflexes |
| Medications | Hypoglycemia | Plantar responses |
| Dietary habits | Hypomagnesemia | Involuntary movements |
| Trauma or poisoning | Asymmetric pulses | |
| Environmental exposure | Bruits | |
| Recent inoculations | Hematologic abnormalities | |
| | Anemia | |
| | Polycythemia | |
| | Hepatomegaly | |

examination should be monitored closely. With any neurologic problem, the progression of deficits is as important as the character of the deficits.

## SYSTEMIC EXAMINATION

Hematologic parameters, vital signs, breathing patterns, cardiac rhythms, and general appearance are all part of the neurologic evaluation. Heart murmurs and arrhythmias are especially relevant in the patient with acutely appearing focal weakness. Emboli from the heart because of arrhythmias or valvular heart disease may produce a stroke.

Cutaneous stigmata, such as hyperpigmented (café-au-lait) or hypopigmented (ash leaf) patches, may denote significant lesions of the central or peripheral nervous system, such as those associated with neurofibromatosis and tuberous sclerosis. A port-wine birthmark over the face may be associated with an intracranial vascular malformation, as in Sturge-Weber syndrome. Profound anemia may account for lethargy, confusion, or even headaches.

Anemia associated with spasticity and loss of position sense may arise with combined systems disease, the neurologic equivalent of pernicious anemia. Electrolyte abnormalities, such as hypomagnesemia, hypocalcemia, or hyponatremia, may induce seizures. Postural hypotension from autonomic nervous system disease, such as that developing with diabetes mellitus, may cause syncope.

## NEUROLOGIC SIGNS

No facet of the patient's examination should be presumed normal unless it is specifically tested. All observations of the patient's characteristics must be treated as potentially significant. An infantile affect, involuntary facial twitch, irregular speech pattern, or peculiar gait should not be dismissed as an idiosyncracy unless it proves to be a longstanding trait with no pathologic basis.

## Mental Status

The patient who looks alert should be specifically questioned about the time, date, location, and situation to determine his or her orientation and recognition of surroundings. Cognitive function should be assessed further with tests of the patient's short-term memory; e.g., recalling 5 items after 5 minutes. If someone is available who can confirm past events, the patient should be asked about activities earlier in the day, earlier in the year, and many years ago. Constructional abilities should be checked by having the patient draw a clockface and a house (Fig. 1-1). Writing and reading ability should be checked with simple phrases and sentences. Any dysarthrias or dysprosodies, abnormalities of speech clarity or rhythms, should be fully described.

Mood swings, loose associations, tangential remarks, and apparent delusions should be observed. The patient must be asked specifically about auditory and visual hallucinations, feelings of persecution, episodes of confusion, blackouts, and convulsions. How the patient perceives his or her neurologic problem is valuable in determining what is causing the neurologic deficit. Patients with right parietal lobe damage often deny left-sided weakness or numbness even when it is profound: some deny that the affected limbs belong to them.

If a problem is detected, the neurologic function that appears to be defective should be tested more extensively. Speech abnormalities should be defined further by checking repetition, comprehen-

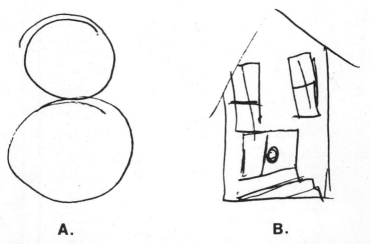

**A.**                              **B.**

FIG. 1-1. A right parietal lobe stroke left the 61-year-old man who drew these (A) circles and (B) house with constructional difficulty. Before his stroke, he was an amateur artist and map maker. After the stroke he could not connect lines or copy drawings. (With permission from Lechtenberg R: *Seizure Recognition and Treatment*. New York, Churchill Livingstone, 1990.)

sion of complex instructions, naming of objects, and more complex reading skills. Because language skills are often related to educational background, the patient's educational history should be sought. Constructional problems may be assessed further by having the patient try to copy complex figures. Whether the patient is right-handed or lefthanded should be determined: a change in hand preference may be the first sign of deteriorating strength or coordination on the dominant side. The patient's ability to name fingers, perform calculations, and perform complex abstractions will help further to define the site and character of the neurologic disease.

## Cranial Nerves

The cranial nerves should be tested individually, with special attention being given to those to which the patient's complaints are referable (Table 1-2).

I. Olfactory. Smell should be tested with materials that have a familiar odor, but are not irritating. Coffee is commonly used; ammonia is too irritating to use. In heavily polluted cities, smell may be defective in otherwise normal individuals because of chemical injuries to the olfactory nerves.

II. Optic. An ophthalmoscopic examination of the eye should be performed and pupillary responses to light and accommodation should be checked in every patient. A pale optic disc from optic atrophy and impaired direct pupillary response to light may be early signs of optic neuritis, an inflammatory disorder of the optic nerve. Elimination of the normal cupping of the optic disc may indicate papilledema, bulging of the optic nerve into the eye caused by increased intracranial pressure. Papilledema is more evident if the margins of

TABLE 1-2.   *Cranial Nerve Examination*

| Nerve | Routine | Poorly Responsive Patient | Probable Coma |
|---|---|---|---|
| I | Smell coffee | None | None |
| II | Check fundi | Check fundi | Check fundi |
|  | Check acuity | Response to threat | Response to threat |
| III | Visual pursuit | Spontaneous eye movements | Spontaneous eye movements |
|  | Pupillary response to light and accommodation | Pupillary response to light | Pupillary response to light |
|  | Optokinetic nystagmus | Oculocephalic reflex | Oculocephalic reflex |
|  |  |  | Caloric response |
| IV | Conjugate eye movements | None | None |
| V | Corneal reflex | Corneal reflex | Corneal reflex |
|  | Jaw movements |  |  |
| VI | Conjugate eye movements | Conjugate eye movements | None |
| VII | Facial movements | Facial movements | Grimacing |
|  | Eye closure | Corneal reflex | Corneal reflex |
| VIII | Auditory acuity | Response to loud noise | Caloric test of labyrinth |
| IX | Gag reflex | Gag reflex | Gag reflex |
| X | Palate retraction | Gag reflex | Gag reflex |
| XI | Sternomastoid and trapezius strength | Head control | None |
| XII | Tongue movements | Tongue position | None |

the optic disc are completely obliterated and hemorrhages and ex-udates have developed on the retina. Brain tumors, meningitis, and intracranial hemorrhages may all produce papilledema.

Visual fields may be checked by testing the patient's ability to count fingers in peripheral and central vision. Perceiving a white-headed pin as it is brought across the visual field is a more sensitive measure of visual fields, but patient cooperation is more likely to be a problem. For the patient who is conscious but unable to co-operate, the blink response to visual threat may be the only test for vision that is feasible. If a problem with vision is likely, acuity and full visual fields should be checked. Bitemporal field defects may be the first sign of a mass, such as a pituitary adenoma, cranio-pharyngioma, or giant aneurysm, pressing on the optic chiasm.

Degenerative changes in the eye, such as the black clumps and yellow swirls of chorioretinitis, may be the most obvious signs of an intrauterine infection such as toxoplasmosis. Pigmentary change in the eye, such as that associated with retinitis pigmentosa, may help explain complaints of deteriorating night vision. Patients with undiagnosed diabetes mellitus may have a proliferative retinopathy causing unexplained loss of visual acuity. Microaneurysms, neo-vascularity, and other changes in the eye may be the first observed signs of this metabolic disease.

III. Oculomotor. Eye movements are dependent on oculomotor (III) as well as trochlear (IV) and abducens (VI) nerve function. Pupillary responses are controlled by parasympathetic fibers carried along the oculomotor nerve and sympathetic fibers originating in the ganglia that lie along the thoracic and cervical spine. The oc-ulomotor nerve also innervates muscles in the eyelid, thereby con-trolling upper eyelid retraction.

Several fiber tracts in the brainstem and cervical spinal cord are instrumental in coordinating eye movements. The medial longitu-dinal fasciculus (MLF) is a major tract coordinating activity in the oculomotor nucleus with that in other ocular motor nerve nuclei. In multiple sclerosis, damage to the MLF produces characteristic disturbances in lateral gaze. The individual with this MLF syndrome has impaired adduction of the adducting eye and an associated nystagmus in the abducting eye when looking to one side.

Normal eye movements include tracking or pursuit movements and step-like or saccadic movements. An object is followed with pursuit eye movements; a series of words is read with saccadic eye movements. Disturbances of either type of movement denote neu-rologic disease. Drawing a striped tape across the visual field will elicit both types of eye movements as the patient follows a line and then makes the visual jump to follow another line. This maneuver demonstrates optokinetic nystagmus, an ocular reflex that may be disturbed by disease at the level of the brainstem or cerebral cortex.

Impaired adduction of the eye, drooping of the eyelid, and pu-pillary unresponsiveness to light may result from an aneurysm on the posterior communicating artery impinging on the oculomotor nerve. Oculomotor palsies with intact pupillary function may occur with ischemic injury to the oculomotor nerve in diabetes mellitus. The irregular Argyll-Robertson pupil of neurosyphilis or diabetes mellitus responds poorly to light, but retains its ability to contract or dilate to accommodate objects placed near or far from the eye. Damage to sympathetic nerves supplying the pupil, such as that occurring with lung cancer impinging on the sympathetic ganglia, may produce a chronically small pupil on the side affected.

If the patient has double vision (diplopia), a piece of red glass or plastic placed over one eye may help determine which muscle is weak. By shining a light at the eyes, the malfunctioning muscle can be identified by the pattern of separation between the red light perceived by the covered eye and the white light perceived by the uncovered eye. The red light will appear to move in the direction the impaired eye is not moving if the red filter is over the weak eye.

Reflex eye movements may be elicited from a stuporous patient by rapidly turning the patient's head to one side or by infusing cold water into one ear. Turning the head elicits the oculocephalic or doll's eye reflex in which the eyes deviate conjugately in the direction opposite the movement. Caloric stimulation of the external ear affects the vestibular organ in the inner ear; cold water infused into the external auditory meatus normally evokes nystagmus in both eyes, the fast component of which is away from the cold ear.

IV. Trochlear. The trochlear nerve innervates the superior oblique muscle. Injury to this nerve may produce a compensatory head tilt. The superior oblique muscle intorts the eye, and so injury to the nerve produces double vision unless the patient compensates by tilting the head. If the oculomotor nerve is damaged and the trochlear nerve is intact, efforts to adduct the eye will produce internal rotation of the globe.

V. Trigeminal. Perception of facial pain is supplied by the ophthalmic, maxillary, and mandibular divisions of the trigeminal nerve. The blink response to corneal irritation is mediated by the first or ophthalmic division of the trigeminal nerve. Sensation over the malar eminences is mediated by the maxillary branch. The mandibular branch supplies the skin over the lower jaw. The temporalis, masseter, and pterygoid muscles of mastication are also controlled by the trigeminal nerve.

VI. Abducens. The abducens nerve innervates the lateral rectus muscle, the muscle responsible for abducting the eye. Abduction of the eye may be impaired if intracranial pressure is increased from a tumor or intracranial hemorrhage.

VII. Facial. The facial nerve controls the muscles of facial expression. Poor facial strength may be inapparent during reflex movement of the face but may become obvious with efforts at voluntarily closing the eyes or smiling. With facial nerve dysfunction, taste and hearing may also be affected because the chorda tympani from the taste buds runs with the facial nerve through some of its course and a branch of the facial nerve innervates the muscle to the stapedius in the middle ear. Damage to the chorda tympani fiber impairs taste. Damage to the stapedius nerve increases sensitivity to noise, a common complaint in patients with idiopathic or Bell's facial palsy.

VIII. Auditory. The auditory nerve carries both acoustic and positional information originating in the cochlea and vestibular elements of the ear. Damage to either the vestibular or acoustic divisions of the nerve usually produces hearing problems because these two elements run so closely together. When hearing is only slightly impaired, word discrimination is usually disturbed. With a tumor, such as a schwannoma, originating on the vestibular division of the nerve, the patient may complain of little more than tinnitus, ringing in the ear.

Tests for differentiating between an acoustic nerve injury and a conductive hearing loss include the Rinne and Weber tests. Both use a low-frequency (256 Hz) tuning fork as the acoustic stimulus. The Weber test helps establish if one ear is more sensitive to sound than the other. It bypasses the tympanic membrane and ossicles of the middle ear by relying on bone conduction of the sound. The vibrating tuning fork is placed on the forehead and the patient reports whether the sound is heard more clearly in one ear than in the other. The normal ear is more sensitive to sound transmitted through the air and amplified by the tympanic membrane and ossicles than to that transmitted to the cochlea through the skull.

The Rinne test also uses this discrepancy between air and bone conduction to help determine whether ear disease involves the neural or conductive elements of the ear. The vibrating tuning fork is left on the mastoid until the vibration is no longer perceptible. If the still vibrating fork is moved to the external auditory meatus, the patient with normal hearing will again hear the vibration. The patient with otosclerosis or other disease of the middle or external ear will perceive the vibration more acutely when the tuning fork is on the mastoid than when it is brought closer to the external auditory meatus. With cochlear or acoustic nerve damage, perception of the tone will be similar whether the fork is on the mastoid or at the external auditory meatus.

IX. Glossopharyngeal. The glossopharyngeal nerve is involved in taste and touch perception about the oropharynx, tongue, and soft palate. Taste may be disturbed and the gag reflex may be lost with glossopharyngeal nerve injury.

X. Vagus. The vagus nerve serves innumerable functions as a regulator of organs ranging from the heart to the stomach, but on neurologic examination little can be perceived of this nerve's activity other than its involvement in the gag reflex. Both reflex and voluntary retraction of the soft palate may be lost with damage to the vagus nerve.

XI. Spinal Accessory. Sternocleidomastoid and trapezius weakness develop with damage to the spinal accessory nerve.

XII. Hypoglossal. Damage to one hypoglossal nerve produces deviation of the tongue toward the weak side. Anterior horn cell disease in the brainstem may produce atrophy and fasciculation of tongue muscles.

## Motor Function

Gait, strength, and tone are readily assessed by having the patient walk, extend the arms in supination, resist the examiner's efforts

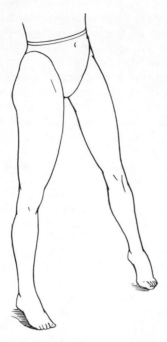

FIG. 1-2. With a spastic hemiparesis, the patient must lift the weak leg at the hip and circumduct it. (With permission from Lechtenberg R: Multiple Sclerosis Fact Book. Philadelphia, F.A. Davis, 1988.)

to overcome individual muscle groups, and allow the examiner to passively move the arms and legs at various joints. Atrophy and involuntary muscle twitches should be looked for as signs of damage to the spinal cord or peripheral nerves. In amyotrophic lateral sclerosis (ALS), muscle bulk may deteriorate over the course of weeks or months and fine, involuntary twitches of the muscles may be evident as the atrophy progresses.

Spasticity, an increased resistance to movement, may be evident even when the patient has no complaints of focal weakness. Spinal cord damage, such as transection of the thoracic spinal cord, produces spasticity below the level of the injury if the corticospinal tracts are damaged. With spastic weakness on one side of the body, the patient may be forced to circumduct the stiff leg at the hip, a gait abnormality commonly seen in patients after a stroke has produced a hemiparesis (Fig. 1-2). Gait abnormalities need not denote weakness: the patient with Parkinson disease may walk with small, shuffling steps and yet have no substantial leg weakness.

### Sensation

Sensation should be specifically checked at least for pain, touch, vibration, and position sense. By having the patient stand on a narrow base, with eyes open and then with eyes closed, position sense may be tested in the legs. This is Romberg's test of position sense; a positive Romberg sign may occur with peripheral neuropathy from diabetes mellitus, as well as from spinal root and cord damage from tabes dorsalis. Individuals with severe cerebellar disease are not able to stand on a narrow base with their eyes open or closed.

The extent of any decreased sensitivity to pain should be mapped out. Common patterns of sensory loss include the glove-and-stocking distribution of diabetic sensory neuropathy and the sensory level of a spinal cord injury. A sensory level should conform to a dermatomal pattern of spinal cord segments. With a peripheral nerve injury, the pattern of sensory loss should conform to the surface area supplied by the peripheral nerve. Injury to the lateral femoral cutaneous nerve produces a patch of decreased sensation over the upper outer aspect of the thigh. Temperature sense and pain perception are often lost concurrently.

More specialized tests of sensory function include two-point discrimination, graphesthesia, and stereognosis. With cerebral cortical damage, these modalities may be severely impaired even without significant loss of pain or touch perception. Two sharp points will feel like one point when they are placed sufficiently closely together. Sufficiently close may be a millimeter or two on the finger tips or a centimeter or two on the back. Asymmetry in two-point discrimination on the two sides of the body suggests damage to the cerebral hemisphere opposite the less sensitive side.

Patients with cerebral cortical damage also have problems discriminating figures traced onto the skin and objects placed into their hands. The number 3 traced on the palm will be unrecognizable. A familiar object, such as a coin, will not be correctly identified when handled by the patient.

### Coordination

Coordination may be tested with fine finger movements, rapid alternating movements (diadochokinesis), and tandem gait (heel-to-toe walking). Coordination of grosser limb movements is evident on having the patient try to reposition the limbs in space without looking at the point at which they arrive (pastpointing) or, while looking, accurately touch a target that shifts in space (dysmetria). Tandem gait, the ability to walk a straight line with heel-to-toe positioning of the feet, tests both coordination and balance.

### Reflexes

Deep tendon reflexes at the biceps, triceps, brachioradialis, patella, and Achilles tendons should always be checked for activity. No activity is rated at 0; hypoactivity is 1 + ; and normal activity is 2 + . Hyperactivity without clonus is 3 + , with transient clonus is 4 + , and with persistent clonus is 5 + . Absent reflexes may develop with spinal root or peripheral nerve injuries. The spinal root injured

TABLE 1-3.   *Deep Tendon Reflexes*

| Reflex | Muscles | Spinal Roots |
|---|---|---|
| Biceps | Biceps | **C5,C6** |
| Triceps | Triceps | C6,**C7**,C8 |
| Brachioradialis | Brachioradialis | C5,**C6** |
| Patellar | Quadriceps femoris | L2,**L3,L4** |
| Achilles | Gastrocnemius and soleus | **S1,S2** |

The spinal root levels in boldfaced type are the predominant ones.

is specific for the reflex that is disturbed (Table 1-3). Absent ankle jerks and unreactive pupils often occur in middle-aged women with the benign reflex disorder called Adie's syndrome.

Firmly stroking the outer margin of the sole of the foot from back to front will elicit a plantar response with flexion of the great toe. Extension of the great toe and fanning of the other toes (Babinski sign) indicates corticospinal tract damage (Fig. 1-3). Reflexes that are normal at one stage of life may resurface with neurologic damage later in life. Infants have a normal grasp reflex that abates with maturation; the same type of traction grasp reflex may reappear with cerebrocortical damage. Sucking and snouting reflexes that are normal in infancy also may develop as pathologic reflexes in adults with cerebrocortical damage. Stroking the palm of the hand may elicit reflex contraction of the ipsilateral triangularis muscle of the chin in the palmomental reflex, a pathologic reflex also associated with brain, especially frontal lobe, damage.

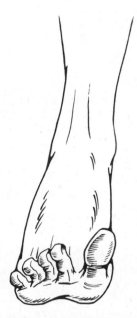

FIG. 1-3. By stroking the lateral edge of the sole of the foot from back to front, the examiner may elicit the characteristic upgoing toe of the Babinski sign if corticospinal tract damage is present.

## COMMON NEUROLOGIC FINDINGS

Some abnormal neurologic findings occur so commonly in the general population that they cannot be considered abnormal if they occur independently of all other signs and do not appear acutely.

### Horner's Syndrome

Unequal pupils may develop with damage to the eye, the sympathetic supply to the iris, or the parasympathetic nerves. If one pupil is smaller than the other and there is decreased facial sweating and apparent lid ptosis ipsilateral to the small pupil, the patient has Horner's syndrome. Horner's syndrome of miosis, ptosis, and anhidrosis occurs with damage to the sympathetic nerves supplying one side of the face. Many pathologic conditions, including apical lung tumors, brainstem strokes, and brain tumors, may interrupt the sympathetic pathway on its way to the eye and face. In many individuals, the damage to the sympathetic system is inconsequential and idiopathic.

A small pupil may also develop as a drug effect, as a consequence of trauma to the eye, or as a symptom of central nervous system infection. One of the best described causes of persistent miosis is neurosyphilis. With CNS infection with Treponema pallidum, the patient may have an Argyll-Robertson pupil. The affected patient can see, often with normal acuity, but the pupil in the affected eye is small, irregular, and unresponsive to light. Unlike the small pupil of Horner's syndrome, the Argyll-Robertson pupil is usually evident in both eyes.

### Adie's Tonic Pupil

Women may have poorly responsive pupils that are tonically dilated. If this is not a drug effect, it may be from an idiopathic syndrome associated with absent Achilles tendon reflexes: Adie's syndrome. Trauma to the eyes must be excluded as a cause of the mydriasis.

### Absent Gag Reflex

Many individuals have poorly reactive or inapparent gag reflexes. If the palate is symmetric and the patient is neither gagging nor aspirating, the hypoactive gag reflex is probably no more than a normal variant.

## SELECTED REFERENCES

Asbury AK, McKhann GM, McDonald WI (eds): Diseases of the Nervous System. Clinical Neurobiology. Philadelphia, W.B. Saunders, 1986.

Barnett HJM, Mohr JP, Stein BM, Yatsu FM (eds): Stoke. Pathophysiology, Diagnosis, and Management. New York, Churchill Livingstone, 1986.

Carpenter MB: Core Text of Neuroanatomy. 3rd Ed. Baltimore, Williams & Wilkins, 1985.

Gilman S, Bloedel J, Lechtenberg R: Disorders of the Cerebellum. Philadelphia, F.A. Davis, 1981.

Gilman S, Winans SS: Manter and Gatz's Essentials of Clinical Neuroanatomy and Neurophysiology. 6th Ed. Philadelphia, F.A. Davis, 1983.

Lechtenberg R: The Multiple Sclerosis Fact Book. Philadelphia, F.A. Davis, 1988.

Lechtenberg R: The Psychiatrist's Guide to Diseases of the Nervous System. New York, John Wiley, 1982.

Medical Research Council: Aids to the Examination of the Peripheral Nervous System. London, Her Majesty's Stationery Office, 1976.

Plum F, Posner JB: The Diagnosis of Stupor and Coma. 3rd Ed. Philadelphia, F.A. Davis, 1980.

Rowland LP (ed): Merritt's Textbook of Neurology. 8th Ed. Philadelphia, Lea & Febiger, 1989.

*Chapter 2*
# Ancillary Tests

The brain, orbits, labyrinths, spinal cord, and associated structures can be visualized with a high degree of resolution by several different neuroimaging techniques. Which technique is appropriate is determined by the character and location of the patient's neurologic problem. Aside from neuroimaging studies, several other tests clarify what damage has occurred in the nervous system. Some look only at function, some at structure, and a few at both. In most cases, information collected from several sources allows an accurate diagnosis to be reached.

## MAGNETIC RESONANCE IMAGING

Magnetic resonance imaging (MRI or MR) uses a high-intensity magnetic field to align many of the protons in the body, a transient electromagnetic pulse (radio wave) to disrupt the alignment, and a radiowave detector to measure local energy changes as the protons realign in the magnetic field. This technique currently assesses little more than the water content of various tissues, but this assessment provides striking anatomic and some physiologic information about the nervous system (Fig. 2-1). Materials with specific properties to enhance contrast where normal structure or physiology has been disrupted may be given to the patient during the study. One of these is gadolinium-DTPA, an agent that ordinarily does not cross the blood-brain barrier but that will accumulate in areas where the blood-brain barrier has been disturbed. Areas with such disturbances include tumor beds, granulomas, and abscesses.

Bone is generally transparent on MR studies, because it has a relatively low water content (Fig. 2-2). Rapidly moving blood also appears largely transparent unless the machine is modified to deal with fluid movement, a modification that has been performed in machines intended to look specifically at blood vessel size and configuration. With gadolinium enhancement, one can identify on the MR scan meningeal spread of tumors, such as that occurring with ependymomas and medulloblastomas, brain tumors seen most often in childhood.

Tumors, infarctions, hemorrhages, and demyelination in the nervous system are easily defined on MR scans. Testing parameters are varied to maximize the clarity of the pictures. The two parameters most often varied are the relaxation time and the repetition rate. The relaxation time is the interval between the interruption of the disruptive radiofrequency pulses and the measurement of electromagnetic waves emitted as realignment in the magnetic field occurs. The repetition rate is the number of times per second that the disruptive radiofrequency wave is applied. Sampling after a brief

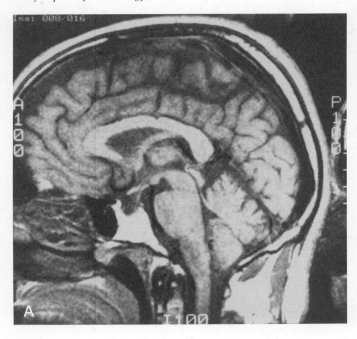

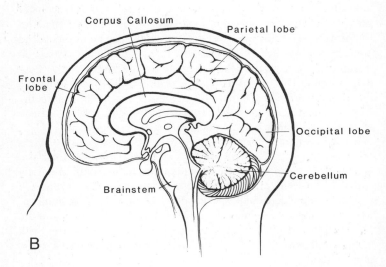

FIG. 2-1. The MR scan (A) provides a saggital view of the head. Some of the obvious structures revealed by the MR scan are labelled in the schematic drawing (B) of a saggital view of the brain. (With permission from Lechtenberg R: Seizure Recognition and Treatment. New York, Churchill Livingstone, 1990.

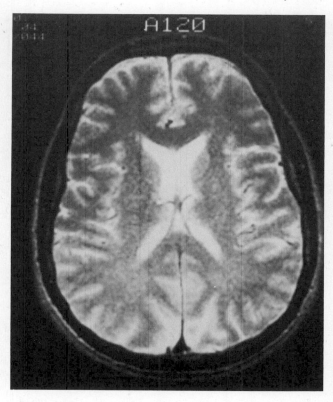

FIG. 2-2. The skull is inapparent on this T2 weighted MR scan of the head. The lateral ventricles appear whiter than other structures in this transverse view of the brain because the MR technique used increases whiteness of the image according to the increasing water content of the tissue.

relaxation time produces an image usually called the T1 view. Longer relaxation times produce the T2 view.

## COMPUTED TOMOGRAPHY

Computed tomography (CT or CAT scanning) uses x-ray absorption to define the density of tissues in the nervous system. Absorption of x-rays by tissues exposed to a low-intensity x-ray beam is measured to calculate the density of the tissue at various locations in the nervous system. CT views are most often obtained along transverse planes through the brain at intervals ranging from a few millimeters to a centimeter (Fig. 2-3). Radiopaque dyes, which do not ordinarily cross the blood-brain barrier, may be administered intravenously to enhance density readings in highly vascular tissue and in tissues with disturbed blood-brain barriers.

Bone is well visualized on the CT scan because of its high density. Blood also contrasts sharply with neural tissue if it is outside blood vessels. This means that acute subdural or epidural hematomas and massive intraventricular or intraparenchymal hemorrhages are ev-

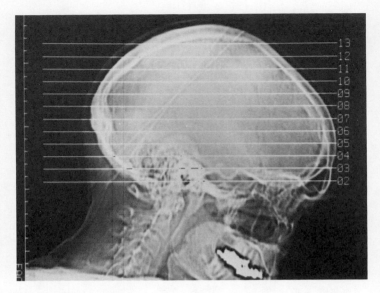

FIG. 2-3. The levels at which CT views will be taken are drawn and numbered on this scout film of the head. CT slices for this study are set at 1-centimeter intervals from the base of the skull to the crown. (With permission from Lechtenberg R: Seizure Recognition and Treatment. New York, Churchill Livingstone, 1990.)

ident on CT scanning. Some tumors, especially those which are calcified, such as meningiomas and oligodendrogliomas, are seen easily with routine CT scanning. Astrocytomas and other lesions with densities close to those of normal neural tissue may require contrast enhancement to better define the lesion. Chronic and subacute subdural hematomas may have densities so close to normal brain tissue that contrast enhancement is needed to improve the resolution of the extraparenchymal mass. Demyelination is usually not well defined by CT scanning, and infarction may only be evident after ischemic changes in the brain have progressed for a day or two.

Both MR and CT scanning are noninvasive tests, but CT scanning may be used with invasive measures, such as intrathecal administration of radiopaque material, to help outline structures impinging on the subarachnoid space. Contrast injection during the CT scan defines large blood vessels in each plane examined by the x-rays. This provides relatively poor views of normal vessels, but it allows demonstration of abnormal vessels, such as giant aneurysms and arteriovenous malformations.

CT slices are routinely performed at 1-cm intervals through the head along transverse planes that capture the bases of the frontal lobes and the posterior fossa in the same view. To obtain higher resolution studies of limited areas, such as the sella turcica or the mastoid air cells, 1-mm slices may be obtained. Such fine slices will reveal microadenomas in the pituitary or hairline basilar skull fractures if such fine lesions are present. CT scanning of the posterior fossa is often disturbed by streak artifacts arising from bone structures close to the neural elements being investigated. MR scanning is not susceptible to this type of artifact and so is especially useful in visualizing nonosseous elements of the posterior fossa.

## ANGIOGRAPHY

Angiography is the radiographic study of blood vessels, whether they be arteries or veins (Fig. 2-4). The technique uses radiopaque dye injected into blood vessels during x-ray study of the vessels. In its simplest form, a catheter is threaded into a vessel, such as the internal carotid, and roentgenograms are obtained during the dye injection. The more selective the vessel catheterized, the more technically difficult the study becomes. Photographic subtraction techniques improve the clarity of vessels travelling through areas of the skull with densities that obscure fine details of the vessel (Fig. 2-5). A negative of the skull is superimposed on a positive of the angiogram to cancel out densities that were present on the roentgenogram before dye injection.

More complex systems, such as digital subtraction angiography (DSA), use computer analysis of x-ray absorption to visualize the injected blood vessels while simultaneously subtracting nonvascular structures that overlie the blood vessels.

MR scanning techniques have been developed that allow selective visualization of the blood vessels in specific parts of the body. Resolution with MR scanning is still poor, but the advantages provided

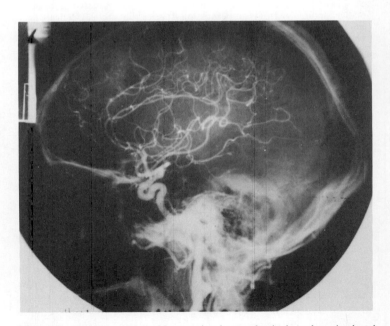

FIG. 2-4. The internal carotid artery has been selectively catheterized and injected to obtain this lateral view of the anterior and middle cerebral arteries.

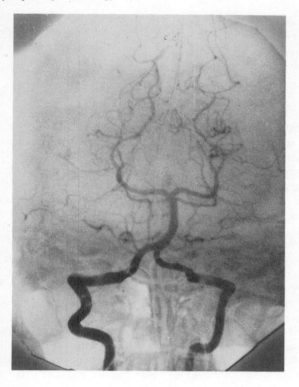

FIG. 2-5. The vertebrobasilar system is well defined on this anterior-posterior projection of the head. The angiogram has been photographically manipulated to subtract much of the bone that would obscure details in the smaller blood vessels. (With permission from Lechtenberg R: Seizure Recognition and Treatment. New York, Churchill Livingstone, 1990.)

by not needing to introduce a catheter into the bloodstream are encouraging further development of this or a similar approach.

Angiography is useful for demonstrating aneurysms, anomalous vessels, and vascular obstructions. Patients with tumors often require angiographic studies to assist the surgeon in planning the approach to the lesion, either for resection or biopsy. With highly vascular lesions, the angiogram may be used to introduce material into the lesion: materials such as small balls or glue, which partially obstruct the vessels feeding the lesion. This embolization simplifies surgical resection by reducing intraoperative bleeding.

## POSITRON EMISSION TOMOGRAPHY

Positron emission tomography (PET) uses positron emitting radionuclides to study metabolic changes in the brain. Computer assessment of the emissions helps localize the emissions to specific areas of the brain. This technique allows consistent measurements of substrate utilization, or at least accumulation, in the brain. By administering a properly tagged substance, the areas in the brain using the material or metabolites of the material may be detected.

This is an investigational tool, currently being used primarily for studies on epilepsy, degenerative disease of the brain, focal brain injuries, and psychologic phenomena. Structural resolution with this technique is extremely poor.

## MYELOGRAPHY

Myelography involves the instillation of radiopaque material into the subarachnoid space to visualize the spinal cord, spinal roots, and adjacent structures. This technique is often combined with CT scanning to enhance visualization of structures about the spinal cord. The subarachnoid dye is usually introduced through a lumbar spinal tap. Cisternal and cervical spine punctures are alternative routes for introducing the material, but placement of a needle at the base of the skull to gain access to the cisterna magna is a relatively complex procedure and should be attempted only by those specifically trained in the technique. Cervical or cisternal punctures are usually necessary when a mass completely obstructs the subarachnoid space and its superior extent must be determined (Fig. 2-6).

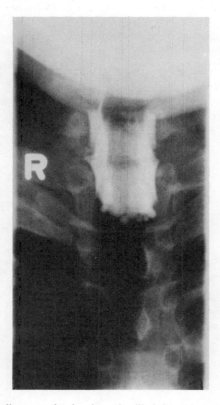

FIG. 2-6. Radiopaque dye has been instilled through a cervical puncture to determine the superior extent of the mass causing signs of spinal cord compression. The column of dye is suspended at the C3–C4 level by a massively herniated intervertebral disc.

Myelography is most useful for identifying intervertebral disc herniation, spinal cord masses, and extra-axial tumors. MR and CT scanning may reveal structures in and about the spinal cord with resolution equal to that of the myelogram, but if no satisfactory diagnosis has been reached with these noninvasive techniques, the myelogram may provide a more definitive answer.

## X-RAY STUDIES OF THE SKULL

Roentgenograms of the plain skull are much less routinely done than in the past, because of the advantages of performing a CT scan. With head trauma, skull x-rays were obtained to look for fractures or indirect evidence of fractures, such as air in the head (Fig. 2-7). A skull fracture is as easily recognized on CT as on roentgenograms of the skull, and the CT provides the additional benefit of demonstrating cerebral contusions or intracranial hemorrhages.

## RADIONUCLIDE STUDIES

Radionuclide studies not using PET scanning techniques are done infrequently. They are still used on rare occasions to look for cere-

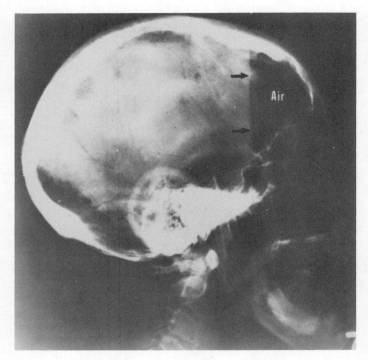

FIG. 2-7. Although no fracture was evident on this skull x-ray, the large collection of air around the brain could only have developed if a fracture had occurred through an area of the skull, such as that overlying the sinuses, which was close to air-filled structures. (From Lechtenberg R: The Psychiatrist's Guide to Diseases of the Nervous System. New York, John Wiley and Sons, 1982.)

brospinal fluid leaks and to look at cerebrospinal fluid flow characteristics. Modifications of obsolete brain scanning techniques with chemical binders, such as amphetamine-like drugs, have had some popularity as inexpensive alternatives to PET scanning. The metabolic information obtained with this single-photon-emission computed tomography (SPECT) scanning is limited and of questionable significance.

## ELECTROENCEPHALOGRAPHY

The electroencephalograph (EEG) records the transient differences in electrical potentials generated by the outer millimeters of cerebral cortex. The placement of electrodes over the scalp and face has been standardized, but the combinations of electrodes used to measure potential differences and the supplementary electrodes used to look at specific areas of cortex vary from institution to institution.

The EEG is usually recorded on continuous sheets of paper that display concurrent recordings from 16 or more different pairs of electrodes. The potential changes appear as oscillations or spikes on the recording. Sharply contoured potential changes lasting less than 80 milliseconds are called spikes. Sharply contoured waves lasting 80 to 200 milliseconds are called sharp waves. Rhythmic changes in potential differences are categorized according to the frequency of the changes. Rhythmic waves at 8 to 12 cycles per second (Hz) are called alpha activity; at 4 to 7 Hz, theta; at 0 to 3 Hz, delta; at 13 to 35 Hz, beta (Table 2-1). Alpha waves normally occur over the back of the head when an individual closes his or her eyes and relaxes (Fig. 2-8). Beta waves are often a consequence of sedative drug use. Theta and delta waves may indicate focal or diffuse cerebral damage. The predominant rhythmic activity is called the background activity. Alpha activity at 8 to 12 Hz is the normal background for relaxed adults.

The EEG was once very useful for localizing structural lesions, such as subdural hematomas and brain tumors, but it has been largely supplanted in assessing the structural integrity of the brain by CT and MR scanning. Its principal application is in the study of seizures and epilepsy. Some types of epilepsy exhibit characteristic EEG patterns. These are discussed in Chapter 5. That a patient has seizures may be demonstrated or supported by visualizing the electrical changes characteristic of the seizure during the EEG or at least by demonstrating spikes, sharp waves, and other phenomena suggestive of an epileptogenic focus (Fig. 2-9).

EEG recordings may be enhanced by manipulating the patient or altering electrode placements. Sleep deprivation, sedation with

TABLE 2-1.  *Brain Wave Patterns*

| Wave | Frequency (Hz) | Significance |
|------|----------------|--------------|
| Delta | 0–3 | ? structural damage |
| Theta | 4–7 | ? structural damage |
| Alpha | 8–12 | normal background |
| Beta | 13–35 | ? drug effect |

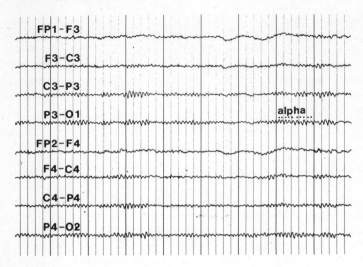

FIG. 2-8. This normal EEG has alpha activity at 10 Hz most evident over the occipital (P3-O1, P4-O2) leads.

chloral hydrate, hyperventilation, and photic stimulation with a strobe light flashed over the closed eyes at various frequencies may elicit epileptiform or epileptogenic phenomena. Nasopharyngeal lead placement may help assess electrical activity on the inner face of the temporal lobe.

Specific diseases may be suggested by the EEG recording, but this study is rarely definitive for establishing a diagnosis. Hepatic or renal encephalopathy may give rise to triphasic waves, recurrent wave forms with three distinct components. With herpes enceph-

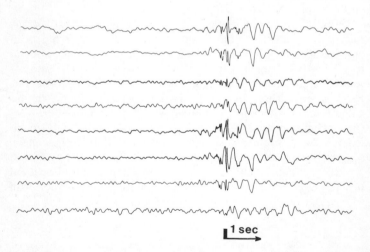

FIG. 2-9. A burst of polyspike and slow-wave activity is evident in all leads of this EEG. It appeared between seizures in this patient with epilepsy. (With permission from Lechtenberg R: Seizure Recognition and Treatment. New York, Churchill Livingstone, 1990.)

alitis, the patient may exhibit temporal lobe abnormalities with sharp waves and spikes originating from one lobe alone or from the most severely affected side and from a mirror focus on the opposite side. Periodic spike or wave discharges may develop with a variety of degenerative and slow-viral illnesses, including subacute sclerosing panencephalitis (SSPE) and Creutzfeldt-Jakob disease.

## EVOKED POTENTIAL STUDIES

Computerized summation of potential changes elicited by auditory, visual, or electrical shock stimuli may provide information on sensory perception and processing. These evoked potential studies use electrodes applied over the spine or the skull to detect consistent deviations from background noise. Summing the response to repetitive stimuli produces a characteristic pattern of waves, with peaks and valleys corresponding to neuronal activity in specific parts of the sensory system. The timing, amplitude, and duration of various components of the evoked potential are altered by damage to components of the sensory system.

Evoked potential changes may be evident long before the patient evidences symptoms. Patients with mild optic neuritis associated with multiple sclerosis exhibit an abnormal visual evoked potential even if they have no visual loss. An acoustic schwannoma associated with neurofibromatosis may produce an abnormal auditory evoked potential long before the patient notices hearing loss or tinnitus.

## ELECTRONYSTAGMOGRAPHY

Electrodes placed about the eyes can record electrical potential changes associated with changes in eye position. The back of the eye is negatively charged in comparison with the front of the eye, so the globe acts as a dipole as it moves. If the patient develops nystagmus for any reason, the record will reveal the character, direction, and intensity of the nystagmus. This electronystagmogram (ENG) is useful in assessing labyrinthine, brainstem, and cerebellar lesions. It provides an objective and reproducible measure of labyrinthine or nervous system disease.

## CEREBROSPINAL FLUID STUDIES

The cerebrospinal fluid is a sensitive indicator of disease in the central nervous system. With bacterial infections affecting the meninges or cerebral cortex, the CSF has a depressed glucose content, with values usually lower than two-thirds the serum glucose level (Table 2-2). With infections, meningeal carcinomatosis, meningeal lymphomatosis, subarachnoid hemorrhage, chemical meningitis, and a variety of other neurologic disorders, the spinal fluid protein exceeds the usual adult maximum of 45 mg/dl. With Guillain-Barré syndrome, the CSF protein content may exceed several hundred mg/dl even though the fluid cell count is largely unchanged from the normal level of 10 mononuclear cells per cmm.

TABLE 2-2.   *Cerebrospinal Fluid Studies*

| Parameter | Normal | Bacterial Meningitis | Viral Meningitis | TB Meningitis | Guillain Barré | Meningeal Carcinomatosis |
|---|---|---|---|---|---|---|
| Opening pressure | Less than 190 mmH$_2$O | Usually increased | Often increased | Often increased | Usually normal | Sometimes increased |
| RBCs/cmm | 0 | 0 | variable | 0 | 0 | 0 |
| WBCs/cmm | 0–10 no polys | >10 some polys | variable | >10 | 0–30 no polys | variable |
| Protein | 15–45 mg/dl | >45 mg/dl | variable | >45 mg/dl | 80–2000 mg/dl | variable |
| Glucose | 2/3 serum content | less than 2/3 serum | variable | less than 2/3 serum | normal | variable |

With subarachnoid hemorrhage, the increase in protein content exceeds that appropriate for blood introduced into the CSF at the time of a traumatic spinal tap. With a normal hematocrit and serum protein, blood introduced by a traumatic spinal tap increases the CSF protein content by only about 1 mg/dl for every 700 red blood cells per cmm of fluid. Blood introduced at the time of a traumatic tap usually forms a clot; blood in the spinal fluid for hours after a subarachnoid hemorrhage does not clot and induces xanthochromia, a yellowish discoloration of the fluid, even if the CSF protein content is only slightly elevated.

With meningeal carcinomatosis or lymphomatosis, the cerebrospinal fluid may contain obviously malignant cells, but more commonly, the fluid reveals little more than an excess of white blood cells or an elevated protein content. The opening pressure may exceed the normal limit of 150 to 190 mm $H_2O$.

Organisms that are difficult to visualize, such as Cryptococcus neoformans, may be sought with antigen-antibody tests of the CSF. More routine organisms should grow in routine culture. Patients at special risk, such as those with AIDS, should have their CSF cultured for fungi, atypical mycobacteria, nocardia, and other organisms usually found only in immunosuppressed individuals. Viral cultures may be appropriate if an epidemic is being followed or if the patient's symptoms suggest a specific agent, but routine screening for a broad spectrum of viral agents is impractical.

## ELECTROMYOGRAPHY AND NERVE CONDUCTION STUDIES

The insertion of needle electrodes directly into muscles provides a record of the electrical changes occurring in the muscle at rest and during voluntary activity. This record is the electromyogram (EMG). It is usually supplemented by using surface electrodes to stimulate nerves supplying the muscles, to evoke activity in sensory nerves, and to record from nerves that have either sensory or motor functions. Measurements of the speed with which an electrical stimulus travels along a nerve is called the nerve conduction (NC) rate.

EMG studies usually identify muscle or anterior horn cell disease. Nerve conduction studies help to identify peripheral nerve lesions. The normal EMG reveals a typical action potential when it is inserted into a minimally active muscle (Fig. 2-10). With maximum

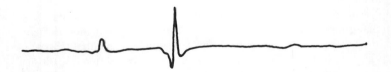

FIG. 2-10. The EMG normally records action potentials that individually resemble the sharply contoured, triphasic element on this tracing.

activity, the combination of muscle fiber action potentials super-imposed on each other obscure the components of the individual potential, producing what is called an interference pattern.

With anterior horn cell disease or other causes of denervation, the muscle exhibits spontaneous activity called fibrillations and fasciculations. Fibrillations are high-frequency, low-amplitude action potentials that produce no overtly apparent muscle activity. Fasciculations are often grossly evident as fragmented muscle twitches of insufficient force to produce movement across a joint. On physical examination, fasciculations may appear as brief undulations of the skin overlying the affected muscle. Other signs of denervation include positive waves, electrical potential waves of inverted polarity that appear during insertion of the EMG needle into the denervated muscle.

Inflammatory muscle disease produces its own characteristic changes in the affected muscle. Action potentials are polyphasic, decreased in amplitude, and less numerous with exertion in muscle with acute or chronic inflammatory disease.

Peripheral nerves with demyelination exhibit slowing of nerve conduction. If the nerve is completely crushed or severed, nerve conduction studies will reveal no transmission of an electrical shock across the block. Retrograde stimulation of nerve fibers is useful in assessing reflex activity.

EMG and NC studies are indispensable for diagnosing amyotrophic lateral sclerosis, polymyositis, diabetic neuropathy, and other diseases primarily affecting the spinal cord, peripheral nerves, or skeletal muscles. These studies cannot differentiate an alcoholic myopathy from a viral polymyositis, but they can establish the existence of generalized muscle disease in a patient abusing alcohol.

## BIOPSY

Biopsy of muscle or nerve tissue may be unavoidable with some diseases. The muscle biopsied is usually one with obvious disease and easy accessibility. Stains for specific enzymes help to classify various myopathies. Deficiencies in mitochondrial enzymes alone account for a large group of myopathic disorders.

The nerve most commonly studied is the sural nerve. This sensory nerve to the heel runs superficially just above the ankle, and damage to it distally produces little more than paresthesias and anesthesia about the heel. The biopsy specimen may reveal demyelination, axonal degeneration, vasculitis in the blood vessels supplying the nerve, abnormal metabolic products in the nerve fibers, or combinations of such abnormalities.

Some unexplained dementias justify brain biopsy, but neuroimaging techniques and EEG studies have made this highly invasive procedure less necessary for the investigation of dementias than was the case several decades ago. Patients with brain tumors still do require biopsy in most cases with only one lesion evident. Direct examination of the tumor tissue allows a rational approach to treatment of the tumor.

## SELECTED REFERENCES

Cohen BH, Bury E, Packer RJ, et al: Gadolinium-DTPA-enhanced magnetic resonance imaging in childhood brain tumors. Neurology *39*:1178, 1989.

Gilman S, Winans SS: Manter and Gatz's Essentials of Clinical Neuroanatomy and Neurophysiology. 6th Ed. Philadelphia, F.A. Davis, 1982.

Lechtenberg R: Seizure Recognition and Treatment. New York, Churchill Livingstone, 1990.

Ross JS, Masaryk TJ, Modic MT, et al: Magnetic resonance angiography of the extracranial carotid arteries and intracranial vessels: A review. Neurology *39*:1369, 1989.

Teasdale GM, Hadley DM, Lawrence A, et al: Comparison of magnetic resonance imaging and computed tomography in suspected lesions in the posterior cranial fossa. Br Med J *299*:349, 1989.

Van der Poel JC, Jones SJ, Miller DH: Sound lateralization, brainstem auditory evoked potentials and magnetic resonance imaging in multiple sclerosis. Brain *111*:1453, 1988.

Vermeulen M, Hasan D, Blijenberg BG, et al: Xanthochromia after subarachnoid haemorrhage needs no revisitation. J. Neurol Neurosurg Psychiatry *52*:826, 1989.

Zanette EM, Fieschi C, Bozzao L, et al: Comparison of cerebral angiography and transcranial Doppler sonography in acute stroke. Stroke *20*:899, 1989.

# Chapter 3
# Unresponsive Patients

The unresponsive patient must be evaluated rapidly to establish the patient's level of consciousness and the basis for the alteration in consciousness. Some causes of unresponsiveness are self-limited and some are lethal. Once the cause of the unresponsiveness is identified, the patient can be treated or observed.

## COMA AND PSEUDOCOMA

The patient with profoundly impaired consciousness who exhibits few if any purposeful reactions to the environment is in coma. Patients who appear to be in coma, but have relatively normal or merely altered consciousness have pseudocoma. Pseudocoma develops with structural brain injuries, encephalitis, metabolic encephalopathy, psychiatric disturbances, and poisoning. Unresponsiveness that is purposefully contrived by the patient is factitious coma.

### Evaluation of the Unresponsive Patient

A variety of methods have been devised to categorize responsiveness. The Glasgow coma scale is routinely used by neurosurgical teams who wish to provide a simple numerical score to characterize the patient's changing level of consciousness with time (Table 3-1). In most cases, it is more valuable to describe fully the patient's apparent level of consciousness, ability to cooperate, response to pain, independent respiratory effort, voluntary and involuntary movements, reflexes, posture, and tone. Changes in these parameters over the course of minutes, hours, or days should be detailed to establish the character and course of the patient's unresponsiveness.

### The Locked-In Syndrome

A lesion in the pons may produce a pseudocoma in which the patient is alert but largely unable to respond to the environment because of loss of voluntary muscle control below the level of the ocular motor nuclei. The patient may exhibit no evidence of consciousness other than purposeful eye movements. This disorder usually occurs with vascular damage to the brainstem. It is generally irreversible and may be a transient state exhibited by a patient with a lethal central nervous system lesion, such as a progressive pontine infarction.

TABLE 3-1.   *Glasgow Coma Scale*

| Testing | Response | Score |
|---|---|---|
| Verbal response | Oriented | 5 |
| | Disoriented, but in context | 4 |
| | Inappropriate words | 3 |
| | Incomprehensible sounds | 2 |
| | Mute | 1 |
| Motor response | Obeys verbal instruction | 6 |
| | Localizes to stimulus | 5 |
| | Withdraws from noxious stimulus | 4 |
| | Postures with arm flexion | 3 |
| | Postures with arm extension | 2 |
| | No response to noxious stimulus | 1 |
| Eye opening | Spontaneous | 4 |
| | With verbal inducement | 3 |
| | With pain | 2 |
| | No voluntary eye opening | 1 |

## Catatonia

Catatonia is a form of unresponsiveness that may develop with severe neurologic or psychiatric disturbances of thought or mood (Table 3-2). The classic signs of catatonia are waxy flexibility, negativism, mutism, posturing, and rigidity. The patient may appear to be awake but is remarkably unresponsive to sensory stimuli, including painful stimuli. The waxy flexibility or catalepsy exhibited by these patients is occasionally striking: limbs placed in awkward postures will return only slowly to more normal postures. Some patients with catatonia exhibit magnetic movements in which limbs move toward light pressure applied to them.

The most common basis for this alteration in responsiveness is schizophrenia, and the most appropriate treatment is antipsychotic medication. Because catatonia may be associated with fever and

TABLE 3-2.   *Causes of Catatonia*

| Nonlethal Catatonia | Lethal Catatonia |
|---|---|
| Schizophrenia | Schizophrenia |
| Hyperpathic akinetic mutism | Viral encephalitis |
| Postictal confusion | Neuroleptic malignant syndrome |
| Subarachnoid hemorrhage | Malignant hyperthermia |
| Viral encephalitis | Neurosyphilis |
| Neurosyphilis | Brainstem stroke |
| Postconcussion syndrome | |
| Parkinsonism | |
| Hyperparathyroidism | |
| Hypothyroidism | |
| Carbon monoxide poisoning | |
| Methioninemia with homocystinuria | |
| Medial temporal lobe lesions | |
| Midbrain injuries | |
| Neurotoxins | |
| Hallucinogens | |
| Tumors of the fornix | |
| Tuberous sclerosis | |
| Medial frontal lobe damage | |
| Systemic lupus erythematosus | |

transient agitation, the schizophrenic with catatonia may look very much like the patient with encephalitis. In fact, several neurologic problems produce catatonic states that worsen or fail to respond when they are managed as psychiatric problems. These neurologic disorders include viral encephalitis and metabolic encephalopathies.

**Metabolic and Structural Causes of Catatonia.**   Hyperparathyroidism with severe hypercalcemia may produce both thought and movement disturbances similar to those exhibited by the schizophrenic with catatonia. Parathyroidectomy with consequent reduction of calcium levels will reverse the catatonia developing with this disorder. A metabolic encephalopathy producing catatonia may also appear in the rare congenital disturbance of homocystine metabolism called homocystinuria with hypermethioninemia. This amino acid disturbance responds somewhat to folate supplements and may be detected by testing the patient's urine reaction to cyanide nitroprusside. Carbon monoxide poisoning may also produce a catatonic-like state, but the damage suffered with this common poison is largely irreversible.

Structural damage to several different parts of the brain may produce transient catatonic states. With generalized head trauma, the patient may have a concussion, subdural hemorrhage, intraventricular bleeding, or subarachnoid hemorrhage, which induces altered responsiveness with a catatonic phase (Fig. 3-1). Frontal lobe, temporal lobe, and midbrain lesions; tumors of the fornix and associated limbic structures; hallucinogens, such as phencyclidine and mescaline; infectious diseases, such as neurosyphilis and parasitic infestations of the brain; and degenerative diseases, such as Pick's disease, all may induce catatonic stupors.

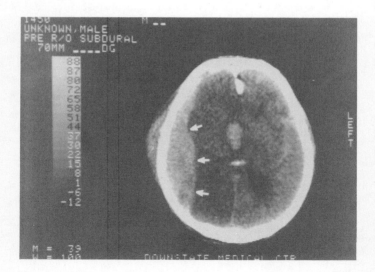

FIG. 3-1. Unresponsiveness similar to catatonia may develop in individuals suffering massive head trauma with associated hemorrhages. This CT scan reveals subdural (arrows) and intraventricular (midline) hemorrhages after massive head trauma. (With permission from Lechtenberg R: Seizure Recognition and Treatment. New York, Churchill Livingstone, 1990.)

**Lethal Catatonia.**   With lethal catatonia, patients develop protracted episodes of unresponsiveness punctuated by periods of extreme agitation, combativeness, disorientation, and delirium. These patients may develop high fevers and severe dehydration if they are not treated with intravenous rehydration. Untreated, they will die from cardiovascular collapse within days or weeks.

Pathologic changes in the brains of patients who die with lethal catatonia are inapparent or limited to some neuronal dropout in the cortex of the frontal lobes. Occasionally, the patients have brainstem injuries, neurosyphilis, viral encephalitis, or the neuroleptic malignant syndrome. Management is largely supportive, with antipyretic treatment and rehydration being essential for survival.

**Neuroleptic Malignant Syndrome.**   Patients receiving haloperidol or phenothiazines, such as fluphenazine, occasionally develop a catatonic state with fever, rigidity, and unresponsiveness as an idiosyncratic reaction to the neuroleptic drugs. This is called the neuroleptic malignant syndrome. Its physiologic basis is unknown. Affected patients often die despite supportive therapy.

## Vegetative States

Chronically unresponsive or poorly responsive patients with established brain damage are in a vegetative state if there is no reversible metabolic, endocrine, or infectious basis for the altered consciousness. The designation vegetative refers to the type of neurologic function that is preserved. Autonomic and reflex actions are intact in the absence of truly purposeful activity. The patient in a vegetative state is not brain dead by current criteria, but may have extensive cerebrocortical damage.

The cerebral cortex may be severely damaged in cardiopulmonary arrest, asphyxia, or head trauma. The patient is apallic if much of the cerebral cortex (pallium) is destroyed. Patients with this and other types of vegetative states may appear awake, blink in response to threat, chew and swallow when food is placed in the mouth, and withdraw limbs from painful stimuli, but these are all reflex activities. In the apallic patient, the EEG does not register any signs of arousal even with painful stimuli. The EEG occasionally is isoelectric, that is, flatline, even when the patient exhibits vegetative responses. By definition, the vegetative state is an irreversible condition.

## Akinetic Mutism

Patients with transient unresponsiveness similar to a vegetative state but with partial or complete resolution of the unresponsiveness are often described as akinetically mute. Patients with akinetic mutism may have lesions in the hypothalamus, brainstem, basal ganglia, or cingulate gyri. An alternative term for this type of reversible unresponsiveness is coma vigile. The patient appears awake, but simply seems unwilling to speak. Superficially, the patient may appear similar to the patient in catatonia, but patients with akinetic

TABLE 3-3. *Characteristics of Catatonia and Akinetic Mutism*

| Catatonia | Akinetic Mutism |
| --- | --- |
| Mutism | Mutism |
| Posturing | Reflex withdrawal from noxious stimuli |
| Waxy flexibility | No retention of imposed postures |
| Rigidity | Spastic or flaccid limbs |
| Intact eye movements | Intact eye movements |
| Apparent vigilance | Apparent vigilance |
| Recall of events during mutism | Amnesia for events during mutism |
| Episodic excitement in some | Episodic excitement in hyperpathic form |
| Hyperthermia in some | Hypersomnia in apathetic form |
| Intact vertical gaze | Paralysis of vertical gaze in some |

mutism do not exhibit the retained postures (waxy flexibility), rigidity, and subsequent recall characteristics of the catatonic patient (Table 3-3).

## BRAIN DEATH

Brain death is an evolving concept that is periodically redefined in both neurologic and legal forums. It designates that state of brain injury that is incompatible with any recovery of cognitive function. Irreversible loss of all apparent cerebrocortical activity is required by all definitions, and irreversible cessation of brainstem function is required by most.

The patients characterized as brain dead must exhibit no response, other than spinal cord reflexes, to any external stimuli. They must have no purposeful or semipurposeful movements, no independent breathing, no eye movements, no corneal responses, no pupillary responses, no oculocephalic or vestibulocephalic reflexes, and no gag reflexes. Attempts to elicit respiratory effort routinely include loading the patient with oxygen and waiting 10 minutes while the patient is disconnected from a ventilator to see whether any breathing movements occur as the arterial $CO_2$ climbs to agreed upon levels. Attempts to elicit eye movements include caloric stimulation of the semicircular canals by infusing ice water into the external auditory meatus.

Specifics of the confirmatory tests used to establish brain death still vary from hospital to hospital. Some require a flatline (isoelectric) EEG recording obtained at unusually high amplification levels, but most have discarded this criterion. All facilities should require that confounding factors, such as hypothermia, drug intoxication, and neuromuscular blockade, are ruled out before deeming the patient brain dead.

## SELECTED REFERENCES

Barnett HJM, Mohr JP, Stein BM, Yatsu FM (eds): Stroke. Pathophysiology, Diagnosis, and Management. New York, Churchill Livingstone, 1986.

Davis RL, Robertson DM (eds): Textbook of Neuropathology. Baltimore, Williams & Wilkins, 1985.

Gilman S, Winans SS: Manter and Gatz's Essentials of Clinical Neuro-anatomy and Neurophysiology. 6th Ed. Philadelphia, F.A. Davis, 1983.

Lechtenberg R: The Psychiatrist's Guide to Diseases of the Nervous System. New York, John Wiley, 1982.

Lechtenberg R: Seizure Recognition and Treatment. New York, Churchill Livingstone, 1990.

Plum F, Posner JB: The Diagnosis of Stupor and Coma. 3rd Ed. Philadelphia, F.A. Davis, 1980.

# Chapter 4

# Syncope

Distinguishing between syncope and seizure activity may be difficult. More characteristic of syncope than of seizures is a consistently brief loss of consciousness. The episode should last seconds, rather than minutes or hours. The patient with syncope does not have any persistent deficits after the loss of consciousness. If premonitory signs occur, they are limited to graying of vision, tinnitus, perioral paresthesias, and shortness of breath.

## CARDIAC AND VASOVAGAL PROBLEMS

Many adults with syncope have cardiac abnormalities or excessively active vasovagal reflexes (Table 4-1). Cardiac arryhthmias may cause syncope by inducing transient hypotension, but hypotension can occur even without an arrhythmia if cardiac activity and vasomotor tone do not reflexively adjust to changes in posture or activity. Excessive autonomic activity may slow cardiac activity inappropriately. This occurs with a hypersensitive carotid sinus, a problem more typically seen in the elderly than in young people.

## VERTEBROBASILAR ISCHEMIA

With insufficient flow to the vertebrobasilar system, the patient may have a variety of complaints referrable to brainstem function and may also experience syncope. The patient with vertebrobasilar insufficiency characteristically has diplopia, vertigo, tinnitus, dysarthria, dysphagia, ataxia, or other signs of vertebrobasilar disease, as well as syncope. Loss of consciousness with poor perfusion of the cerebral hemispheres is highly improbable: infarction of much of the cerebral cortex in one hemisphere usually does not produce a loss of consciousness.

## ORTHOSTATIC HYPOTENSION

Orthostatic hypotension with syncope may develop on standing if cardiac activity does not respond to the shifts in blood volume that occur with assuming an upright position. Changes in posture also require changes in vascular tone to maintain cerebral perfusion. With a substantial drop in blood pressure on assuming an upright posture, the patient will faint. Several neurologic disorders, including Shy-Drager syndrome and Parkinson disease, may lead to orthostatic hypotension (Table 4-2). The most common element in most problems leading to orthostatic hypotension is a failure of the sympathetic division of the autonomic nervous system.

TABLE 4-1.   *Causes of Syncope*

Hysterical unresponsiveness
Hyperventilation syncope
Orthostatic hypotension
Cardiac arrhythmias
Seizures
Subclavian steal syndrome
Transient ischemic attacks
Hypersensitive carotid sinus
Basilar impression

Sympathetic activity is responsible for regulating arteriolar tone, venomotor tone, myocardial contractility, and cardiac rate. Neurologic diseases causing substantial sympathetic damage also usually produce problems with bowel function, sweating, and sexual function. This constellation of problems is often apparent in individuals with severe diabetes mellitus, amyloidosis, or thiamine deficiency.

The widespread use of antihypertensive agents causes iatrogenic hypotension in sensitive or overmedicated individuals. The elderly are especially susceptible to excessive sympathetic blockade with associated orthostatic hypotension and syncope. Orthostatic hypotension not readily traced to an iatrogenic, degenerative, metabolic, nutritional, cardiac, or hematologic basis is called primary.

Primary orthostatic hypotension is assumed to arise from defective central nervous system regulation of autonomic function. Typical of primary orthostatic hypotension is the absence of premonitory signs, such as diaphoresis and bradycardia, presumably because both cholinergic and adrenergic central nervous system activity are defective.

## HYPERVENTILATION SYNCOPE

Young adults who have no apparent cardiac disease and are not receiving medications, such as guanethidine, which might interfere with autonomic activity, may have syncope with hyperventilation. The patient breathes inappropriately rapidly as a response to stress or depression. Hyperventilation produces a respiratory alkalosis as carbon dioxide is cleared from the blood. Syncope occurs as the

TABLE 4-2.   *Causes of Orthostatic Hypotension*

Volume depletion from blood loss
Cardiac disease
Addison disease
Diabetes mellitus
Amyloidosis
Thiamine deficiency
Parkinson disease
Shy-Drager syndrome
Tabes dorsalis
Combined systems disease
Antihypertensive medication
Prolonged bedrest
Primary orthostatic hypotension

premonitory signs of graying vision, tingling about the mouth, and paresthesias in the hands increase the patient's agitation and aggravate the hyperventilation. As the respiratory alkalosis worsens, the patient transiently loses consciousness. With the loss of consciousness, postural tone is lost and the patient falls if he or she is standing. Within a few seconds of the loss of consciousness, the respiratory alkalosis corrects itself and the patient recovers with full recall of the events leading to the syncope. The respiratory alkalosis may be blunted by having the patient breathe into a closed container when he or she feels faint, thereby increasing the carbon dioxide content of the inhaled air.

## BASILAR IMPRESSION

Syncope occasionally develops if the patient has malformations at the base of the skull. This may occur in association with cervical spine abnormalities, as in the Klippel-Feil syndrome, or with cerebellar malformations, as in the Chiari malformations. Affected individuals may report dizziness, tinnitus, blurred or double vision, altered hearing, and syncope on neck extension. Syncope may result from vertebrobasilar obstruction with changes in head position.

## SELECTED REFERENCES

Asbury AK, McKhann GM, McDonald WI (eds): Diseases of the Nervous System. Clinical Neurobiology. Philadelphia, W.B. Saunders, 1986.

Auer RN, Siesjo BK: Biological differences between ischemia, hypoglycemia, and epilepsy. Ann Neurol 24:699, 1988.

Barnett HJM, Mohr JP, Stein BM, Yatsu FM (eds): Stroke. Pathophysiology, Diagnosis, and Management. New York, Churchill Livingstone, 1986.

Lechtenberg R: The Psychiatrist's Guide to Diseases of the Nervous System. New York, John Wiley, 1982.

Lechtenberg R: Seizure Recognition and Treatment. New York, Churchill Livingstone, 1990.

Mooradian AD: Diabetic complications of the central nervous system. Endocr Rev 9:346, 1988.

Rowland LP (ed): Merritt's Textbook of Neurology. 8th Ed. Philadelphia, Lea & Febiger, 1989.

# Chapter 5
# Transient Neurologic Signs

Neurologic signs and symptoms that appear abruptly and resolve over the course of minutes or hours usually develop with transient ischemia or seizure activity. The pattern of neurologic changes, the clinical setting in which the events occur, and the long-term sequelae of the neurologic events help determine whether ischemia or seizure activity is the basis for the deficits. Occasionally, expanding lesions, such as brain tumors or chronic subdural hematomas, may produce transient signs and symptoms, but the character of the underlying lesion usually becomes evident within days or weeks as the lesion progresses and deficits persist.

## TRANSIENT ISCHEMIC ATTACKS

A transient ischemic attack (TIA) is an episode of neurologic deficit caused by insufficient blood flow to a limited part of the central nervous system (CNS). By definition, the deficits appear abruptly and resolve completely in less than 24 hours. The character of the deficits is determined by the area of the CNS that is ischemic. Implicit in the term transient ischemia is the assumption that irreversible neurologic damage has not occurred, but some individuals with clinically transient deficits have identifiable, though silent, infarction of brain or spinal cord tissue. The impairment of blood flow is presumed to be insufficient or too short-lived to produce permanent neuronal injury or loss. Episodes in which the deficits appear to resolve completely after an interval longer than 24 hours are called reversible ischemic neurologic deficits (RINDS).

TIAs are followed by strokes within a few weeks in as many as one fourth of cases. Because they are so strongly correlated with strokes, investigation and treatment of the attacks must be done quickly. The most easily corrected problems are those associated with platelet or clot emboli originating on diseased heart valves or ulcerated atherosclerotic plaques. Because these emboli are preventable with anticoagulation, many physicians feel obliged to start the victim of a TIA on anticoagulants, such as heparin and warfarin, as soon as possible. How long the anticoagulation should be continued is highly controversial, with treatment formulas varying from weeks to years.

### Pathogenesis of TIAs

Impaired flow to parts of the brain may develop with local disease or with remote disease producing local problems (Table 5-1). Cerebrovascular disease from atherosclerosis in either the major vessels or their terminal branches is currently the most common cause of TIAs in the United States. Vascular disease associated with hyper-

TABLE 5-1.   *Diseases Associated with TIAs*

| |
|---|
| Atherosclerotic cerebrovascular disease |
| Chronic hypertension |
| Diabetes mellitus |
| Valvular heart disease |
| Carotid or vertebrobasilar artery occlusion |
| Cervical spondylosis |
| Complicated migraine |
| Subclavian steal |
| Anemia |
| Polycythemia |
| Sickle cell disease |
| Hyperlipidemia |

tension is also common, but bleeding from Charcot-Bouchard aneurysms and other complications of hypertensive cerebrovascular disease are more likely to produce persistent, rather than transient, neurologic deficits. With diabetes mellitus, patients are at greatly increased risk of atherosclerotic cerebrovascular disease and consequently face an increased risk of TIAs and strokes.

Any problem disturbing the normal viscosity of blood, whether it be erythrocyte deformation in sickle cell disease or hyperlipidemia in cholesterol receptor disorders, may produce TIAs. Profound anemia occasionally produces ischemic attacks, but this clinical situation usually does not present diagnostic problems. With severe cervical spine disease, the vertebral arteries may be impinged on by boney spurs and ridges as they travel through the transverse processes of the cervical spine. Narrowing of these vessels may ultimately produce vertebrobasilar TIAs. Alternatively, vascular anomalies or occlusions in the major vessels arising from the aorta may shunt blood away from the brainstem to supply the subclavian artery. When the patient makes extra demands on the affected arm, shunting of blood away from the vertebrobasilar system may be substantial enough to be symptomatic. This is called a subclavian steal syndrome.

## Symptoms of TIAs

The types of neurologic problems observed during any TIA are determined by the vessels involved. Middle cerebral artery ischemia may produce hemiparesis, hemisensory deficit, and aphasia if the artery to the dominant hemisphere is affected. Ophthalmic artery obstruction produces transient blindness, that is, amaurosis fugax, in one eye. Posterior cerebral artery involvement causes transient visual field defects or complete blindness. Vertebrobasilar attacks usually produce vertigo, slurred speech, ataxia, diplopia, facial weakness, or other signs of brainstem and cerebellar dysfunction. Vertigo or dizziness occurring without other signs of posterior fossa disease are usually not from vertebrobasilar insufficiency.

## Investigation of TIAs

Patients with TIAs should be investigated for valvular heart disease with echocardiography. If the heart is not the source of emboli producing the TIAs, angiography may be appropriate. Whether to perform an angiogram depends in part on whether the patient is considered a surgical candidate. For most individuals, the finding of an ulcerated plaque in the carotid artery on the side corresponding to the side of the brain that appears to be having the TIAs is sufficient reason to perform a carotid endarterectomy. If the patient is not a surgical candidate because of age or associated conditions, angiography may be inappropriate.

## Management of TIAs

Nonsurgical approaches to TIAs include anticoagulation with heparin and warfarin. Patients with chronic hypertension, coagulopathies, ulcers, diverticulosis, and other conditions increasing the risk of bleeding should not be started on heparin or warfarin. Some individuals have fewer TIAs if they receive aspirin or other anti-platelet-aggregating agents.

Managing TIAs with endarterectomy has been disappointing. Increasingly critical studies have revealed that only a small segment of the population with TIAs profits from resection of carotid artery plaques. No apparent benefit accrues from performing endarterectomies on the vertebrobasilar system. Regardless of how patients with TIAs are managed, about one fourth eventually die of myocardial infarctions or arrhythmias.

## SEIZURES AND EPILEPSY

Seizures are episodes of disorganized electrical activity in the brain producing transient neurologic deficits. These deficits may include loss of consciousness, involuntary movements, abnormal sensory perceptions, focal weakness, cognitive disorders, affective changes, autonomic dysfunction, or other neurologic signs and symptoms. The tendency to have recurrent seizures is called epilepsy. Some forms of epilepsy occur with very specific patterns of phenomena and are legitimately considered syndromes. Others exhibit numerous features that are idiosyncratic to the patient who is affected.

## Seizure Types

Seizures usually occur in one of two forms, generalized and partial (Table 5-2). Partial seizures may generalize secondarily. Some seizure types routinely have premonitory signs, called the aura. The obvious seizure phenomena associated with either generalized or partial seizures are called the ictus. Either type of seizure may leave the patient with transient neurologic deficits after the obvious seizure episode. These are called postictal deficits. Phenomena occurring between the postictal period of one seizure and the aura of the next seizure are designated the interictal phenomena.

**Generalized Seizures.** In the generalized seizure, electrical activity recorded from the cortex abruptly changes, often with spikes

TABLE 5-2.   *Seizure Types*

| Generalized | Partial |
|---|---|
| Tonic-clonic (Grand mal) | Complex |
| Absence (Petit mal) | Simple motor (Focal motor) |
| Atypical absence | Simple sensory (Focal sensory) |
| Tonic | Secondarily generalized |
| Clonic | |
| Clonic-tonic-clonic | |
| Atonic | |
| Myoclonic | |
| **Unclassified (Neonatal, etc.)** | |

arising simultaneously from many different parts of the cortex. The patient invariably loses consciousness, and in some types of generalized seizures, the patient loses postural tone. If tone is not lost and the patient has little more than altered consciousness, the seizure may fulfill the criteria for a generalized absence attack. These absence attacks last seconds and are associated with a characteristic EEG pattern of 3-per-second spike-and-wave combinations (Fig. 5-1).

Generalized seizures in which the patient loses postural tone and develops tonic and clonic contractions of major muscle groups are called generalized tonic-clonic seizures. These last seconds to minutes and are often associated with a period of confusion and weakness after the seizure, called the postictal period. The postictal period may last minutes or hours. This postictal period is not a facet of generalized absence seizures, but may occur with some types of partial seizures.

**Partial Seizures.**   Partial seizures start in a limited part of the cerebral cortex and either remain restricted to a fairly limited area or generalize secondarily to the rest of the cortex. They are either

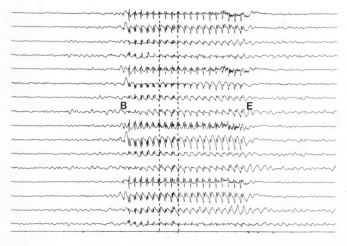

FIG. 5-1. The child from whom this EEG was taken had a generalized absence attack lasting 7 seconds (B to E). During each second of the seizure (interval between dashed lines), 3 spike-and-slow-wave complexes appeared in each lead of the EEG. (With permission from Lechtenberg R: Epilepsy and the Family. Cambridge, Harvard University Press, 1984.)

complex or simple. The simple seizures usually affect one neurologic faculty, such as strength in a limb or sensation over part of the body, at a time. Consciousness is not lost with simple partial seizures.

With complex partial seizures, consciousness is always lost (Table 5-3). The patient usually has an aura. The ictus of the seizure, that is, the interval during which highly typical seizure phenomena occur, is usually longer than a minute and rarely less than 10 seconds. The complex partial seizure often arises in the temporal lobe and may generalize secondarily to a tonic-clonic seizure (see Fig. 5-2). It often leaves the patient with transient postictal deficits. During the ictus, the EEG commonly exhibits unilateral or bilateral temporal or frontal lobe spike discharges. Between obvious seizures, the EEG may show focal spikes or sharp waves or be completely normal.

The simple partial seizure may consist of little more than an aura. The patient never loses consciousness during this type of seizure, and the seizure itself usually lasts less than 30 seconds (Table 5-3). As with the complex partial seizure, the simple partial seizure may generalize to a tonic-clonic seizure. The affected individual only rarely has any postictal deficits. The EEG usually exhibits focal-spike or sharp-wave discharges over the affected cortex during the ictus. These may also be evident interictally.

### Etiology of Seizures

Seizures arise from injuries to or irritation of the cerebral cortex. In many people, the cause of this injury or irritation is not evident, in which case, the seizures are cryptogenic. In many instances, the cause of the cortical problem is evident, such as after massive head trauma or in acute meningoencephalitis. When the seizures arise as part of a distinct epileptic syndrome, the basis for which may be unknown but the course and characteristics of which are fairly stereotyped, the disorder may be considered idiopathic but not truly cryptogenic. The basis for the syndrome is unknown, but the basis for the seizures is the epileptic syndrome.

Seizures occurring shortly after birth may be from intrauterine infections, metabolic disorders, subarachnoid hemorrhage, asphyxia, or other neurologic calamities to which the neonatal brain is vulnerable (Table 5-4). Infants and very young children may develop isolated seizures in association with high fevers, so-called febrile seizures, but these seizures do not predict that the child will exhibit epilepsy later in life unless they are associated with focal neurologic signs, intellectual impairment, or a family history of epilepsy. The inconsequential febrile seizures are called simple; those associated with a higher risk of epilepsy are called complex (Table 5-5). A more sinister form of seizures that occurs in infants is the infantile spasm. The infant exhibits myoclonic jerks and other types of irregular movements usually associated with a profoundly abnormal, high-amplitude EEG pattern arising from the entire cerebral cortex.

Adolescents and young adults are especially susceptible to seizures associated with substance abuse, but in either age group the possibility of an epileptic syndrome or underlying structural brain

TABLE 5-3. *Characteristics of Different Seizure Types*

| | Seizure Type | | | |
|---|---|---|---|---|
| Characteristic | Partial Complex | Generalized Absence | Generalized Tonic-Clonic | Partial Simple |
| Aura | Usually | Never | Sometimes | Rarely |
| Loss of consciousness | Always | Always | Always | Never |
| Automatisms | Commonly | Rarely | No | No |
| Postictal confusion | Usually | Never | Usually | No |
| Duration | Minutes | Seconds | Minutes | Seconds to minutes |

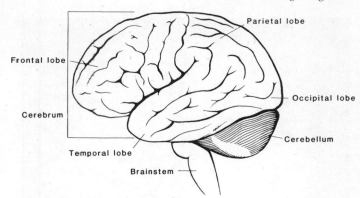

FIG. 5-2. Complex partial seizures often arise in the temporal lobe. (With permission from Lechtenberg R: Epilepsy and the Family. Cambridge, Harvard University Press, 1984.)

TABLE 5-4.  *Causes of Seizures*

| In Adults | In Infants |
| --- | --- |
| Cryptogenic | Intrauterine infection |
| Head trauma | Fever |
| Drug use | Trauma |
| Infection | Poisoning |
| Hemorrhage | Infection |
| Stroke | Hemorrhage |
| Tumor | Vascular malformation |
| Vasculitis | |
| Parasites | |
| Poisoning | |

lesion should not be overlooked. Acquired immune deficiency syndrome (AIDS) is an increasingly common problem in both newborns and young adults and must be considered as a basis for seizure activity at any age. The human immunodeficiency viruses (HIVs) may cause seizures by directly damaging the cortex or by enabling opportunistic infections to establish themselves in the brain. Adults over 30 years of age developing seizures for the first time must be presumed to have a structural brain lesion, such as a brain tumor

TABLE 5-5.  *Febrile Seizures*

| Simple | Complex |
| --- | --- |
| 1 to 5 years of age | Before 1 year of age |
| Generalized | Partial simple or complex |
| Less than 15 minutes | More than 15 minutes |
| Only family member affected | Other family members with seizures |
| Normal neurologic exam | Persistent neurologic deficits |
| Treatment | |
| Antipyretics (e.g., acetaminophen) | Antiepileptics (e.g., phenobarbital) |
| Alcohol rubs | Manage infection or other treatable cause |
| Cooling baths | |

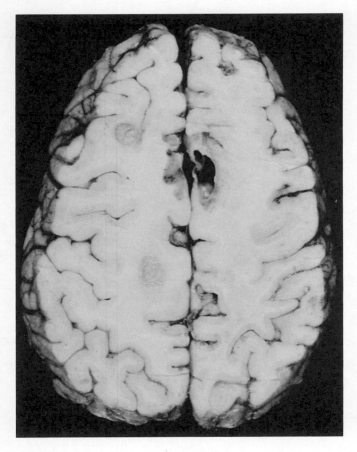

FIG. 5-3. The circular punched-out lesions on the left side of this brain are abscesses. Such lesions often produce seizures in affected individuals.

or abscess, or a CNS infection, such as pneumococcal meningitis, until proven otherwise (Fig. 5-3). The elderly may develop seizures in association with strokes or degenerative diseases, such as Alzheimer's disease, but they too should be investigated for treatable causes of seizures.

### Investigation of Seizures

The investigation of the patient with a seizure disorder should routinely include an EEG and CT or MR scan. The neuroimaging studies may reveal unreported head trauma in the very young or the very old. The EEG may suggest a focal problem in patients with more obvious diffuse disease. The patient with diffuse degenerative changes from Alzheimer's disease may have an epileptogenic focus from an unsuspected astrocytoma.

If there is reason to suspect a CNS infection, cerebrospinal fluid must be cultured. Investigations should be undertaken aggressively

TABLE 5-6. *Drug Use Associated with Seizures*

| With Use | With Withdrawal |
|---|---|
| Cocaine | Alcohol |
| Ampetamines | Barbiturates |
| Methaqualone | |
| Aminophylline | |

in very young children with seizures, fever, and neck stiffness because the risk of meningitis is relatively high and the lethality of infections is great. The child with recurrent ear infections and new-onset seizure activity should have neuroimaging studies done to look for brain abscess before a lumbar puncture is performed. The risk of herniation with a lumbar puncture is substantial when a child has a posterior fossa abscess.

Because some drugs, including cocaine and amphetamines, precipitate seizures when their levels in serum are rising, drug screens are increasingly valuable in the investigation of new-onset seizure disorders (Table 5-6). Alcohol and barbiturates should be screened for along with the stimulant drugs, because these largely depressant drugs may evoke seizures as a withdrawal effect. As the alcohol or barbiturate levels fall, the individual may have seizures even if he or she does not have epilepsy.

All patients should have serum electrolytes, including magnesium and calcium, checked along with determinations of serum glucose levels. Hemoglobin disorders, such as sickle cell and thalassemia, should be screened for if more obvious causes of brain disease are not apparent. Extensive metabolic studies are appropriate in infants with nonfebrile seizures.

### Control of Seizures

Antiepileptic drugs are usually needed to control seizures, unless the cause of the seizure is obviously reversible or self-limited. The child with simple febrile seizures usually requires nothing more than antipyretic treatment to control the seizures (see Table 5-5). Patients with alcohol withdrawal seizures may respond satisfactorily to oral benzodiazepine treatment, which is not usually effective for controlling seizures arising from other causes. In most cases, however, an effective antiepileptic agent must be administered and continued for months or years after the first seizure occurs.

**Neonatal Seizures.** In the neonatal period, investigation and control of the seizure must be completed rapidly to minimize the risk of permanent damage to the infant. Glucose, calcium, and magnesium must be supplemented if they are deficient (Table 5-7). Pyridoxine should be administered even if it does not appear to be deficient. If the seizures are not arising from a readily correctable problem, such as hypocalcemia, phenobarbital should be used as an antiepileptic measure.

**Drug-Related Seizures.** Individuals with drug-related seizures may need antiepileptics even though the cause of the seizures is reversible

TABLE 5-7.  *Management of Neonatal Seizures*

IV $D_{25}W$ solution at 0.5–1.0 g/kg if hypoglycemic
5% calcium gluconate IV at 200 mg/kg if hypocalcemic
50% magnesium sulfate IM at 0.2 ml/kg if hypomagnesemic
Trial of pyridoxine IV 50 mg with EEG monitor
Emergency lumbar puncture
For Persistent Seizures
Loading dose of phenobarbital IV 15 mg/kg
Phenobarbital IV 5 mg/kg up to maximum of 40 mg/kg
Loading dose of phenytoin IV 10 mg/kg
Additional doses of phenytoin up to maximum of 20 mg/kg
Support blood pressure and breathing
Monitor serum antiepileptic levels
Intravenous antibiotics for meningoencephalitis

(Table 5-8). Antiepileptics protect the individual from status epilepticus, potentially lethal, unremitting seizure activity. Those patients requiring antiepileptics are usually managed most effectively with phenobarbital, even though withdrawal from this barbiturate must be done gradually to avoid seizures related to use of this medication.

**Drug Doses.**  The choice and dose of antiepileptic medication is determined by the patient's age, size, and seizure type (Table 5-9). Serum levels of the drug administered should be monitored periodically to ascertain how the individual handles the drug given, but the dose of drug advisable for any individual is the amount needed to control seizures and minimize drug side effects. Therapeutic levels are published for each of the drugs used as antiepileptics, but what is therapeutic for most of the population need not apply for the individual patient (Table 5-10). If the therapeutic serum level is ideal for the individual, it may still require an oral dose of drug greater or less than that recommended for the general population. A variety of systemic problems may interfere with the normal absorption, metabolism, binding, and excretion of antiepileptic drugs. Liver and kidney disease are especially likely to affect several of these parameters, and dosage adjustments must be made if problems with these organs are evident.

If seizures cannot be controlled with the drug of choice or the drug of choice produces unacceptable side effects at the dose needed

TABLE 5-8.  *Management of Seizures Related to Substance Abuse*

| | |
|---|---|
| Alcohol | Detoxify with chlordiazepoxide 25 to 100 mg 4 to 6 times daily PO |
| | Thiamine 100 mg IM or IV for at least 3 days |
| Barbiturates | Load with phenobarbital 200 mg IV |
| | Follow up with phenobarbital 100 mg IV or PO on following 2 days |
| | Taper by 35 mg daily IV or PO over next 3 days |
| Cocaine | Monitor and stabilize autonomic function |
| | Special attention to cardiac rhythm |
| | Avoid antiepileptics unless multiple seizures occur |
| | Phenobarbital 100 mg IV for 2 days if seizures persist |
| | Taper phenobarbital IV or PO over 3 days |
| Amphetamines | Same procedure as for cocaine |
| Methaqualone | Same procedure as for cocaine but without excess cardiac precautions |

TABLE 5-9.  *Antiepileptic Dosage for Children*

| Drug Name | Brand Name | Usual Dose (mg/kg/day) | Serum Half-life (hrs) |
|---|---|---|---|
| Phenobarbital | — | 3–5 | 30–50 |
| Phenytoin | Dilantin | 4–7 | 3–11 |
| Primidone | Mysoline | 10–25 | 6–8 |
| Carbamazepine | Tegretol | 20–30 | 6–16 |
| Valproate | Depakote | 15–60 | 4–14 |
| Clonazepam | Klonopin | 0.01–0.20 | 16–60 |
| Ethosuximide | Zarontin | 20–40 | 24–30 |

to control seizures, an alternative drug must be used. Only one drug should be used to control seizures, unless trials with a variety of individual drugs have failed and a combination of two drugs provides good seizure control without producing unacceptable side effects.

**Drugs of Choice.**   For generalized tonic-clonic seizures, valproate (divalproex sodium or valproic acid), carbamazepine, and phenytoin are usually effective, but the preferred drug is valproate for individuals over 10 years of age (Table 5-11). Problems with hepatic reactions in children under 2 years of age and much more rarely in individuals between 2 and 10 years of age have made valproate less preferred in this age group. Complex partial seizures are also often controlled with any of these three drugs, but carbamazepine is the current drug of choice. Generalized absence seizures in children respond to ethosuximide or valproate, but concerns about liver problems in very young children have made ethosuximide the drug of choice for this seizure type. Myoclonic seizures often respond to clonazepam. Focal motor (simple partial motor) seizures are usually managed with carbamazepine or phenytoin. Infantile spasms may respond to adrenocorticotropic hormone (ACTH), but even with control of these seizures, the outlook for the child in terms of intellectual function or even survival is poor.

**Seizure Surgery.**   Patients refractory to antiepileptic medications may benefit from brain surgery. Techniques currently employed include resection of seizure foci and division of the corpus callosum. Seizure foci are usually identified by recordings from the surface of the cortex and by recordings from implanted electrodes. Criteria for subjecting an individual to seizure surgery are highly restrictive because many patients with focal neurologic deficits, psychiatric

TABLE 5-10.  *Antiepileptic Dosage for Adults*

| Drug Name | Brand Name | Usual Dose (mg/kg/day) | Therapeutic Level (μg/ml) | Days to Steady State | Serum Half-life (hrs) |
|---|---|---|---|---|---|
| Carbamazepine | Tegretol | 10–25 | 6–12 | 3–6 | 8–19 |
| Valproate (Valproic acid) | Depakote Depakene | 10–70 | 50–100 | 2–4 | 7–17 |
| Phenytoin | Dilantin | 4–10 | 10–20 | 5–10 | 22–40 |
| Ethosuximide | Zarontin | 20–40 | 40–100 | 6–12 | 50–60 |
| Primidone | Mysoline | 10–25 | 6–12 | 1–5 | 8–16 |
| Phenobarbital | — | 1–5 | 15–35 | 16–21 | 50–96 |
| Clonazepam | Klonopin | .03–.10 | .013–.072 | — | 16–60 |

TABLE 5-11.   *Drugs of Choice*

| Seizure Type | First Choice | Alternatives |
|---|---|---|
| Complex partial | Carbamazepine | Valproate<br>Phenytoin |
| Simple partial | Carbamazepine | Phenytoin |
| Generalized tonic-clonic | Valproate | Carbamazepine<br>Phenytoin |
| Generalized absence | Ethosuximide | Valproate<br>Clonazepam |
| Infantile spasms | ACTH | Corticosteroids<br>Valproate<br>Phenobarbital |
| Complex febrile | Phenobarbital | Valproate<br>Primidone |

problems, or cognitive impairment fail to profit substantially from this highly invasive procedure.

## PSEUDOSEIZURES

Episodes of apparently altered consciousness or altered responsiveness that resemble seizures are called pseudoseizures. Episodes purposely or subconsciously contrived to resemble true seizures are called factitious seizures. Many patients with true seizures also have factitious seizures; simply determining whether an individual has epilepsy does not establish that an individual seizure is authentic or factitious. Determining whether a seizure is real or not is important in deciding whether the patient's antiepileptic regimen is sufficient.

Seizure-like phenomena that present diagnostic dilemmas include paroxysms of shuddering in newborns, esophageal reflux and breathholding spells in infants, and syncope in adults. A variety of sleep-related phenomena, including somnambulism, somniloquy, bruxism, and night terrors, are superficially reminiscent of seizures, but EEG recordings obtained during sleep should clarify the basis for the suspicious behavior. More obviously psychiatric disorders, such as panic attacks, dissociative disorders, and psychoses, may be much more difficult to distinguish from partial seizure disorders. Ambulatory EEG monitoring may be useful, but additional neurologic testing, including CT or MR scanning, is appropriate for any new-onset cognitive or affective disorder.

## STATUS EPILEPTICUS

Recurrent seizure activity uninterrupted by intervals during which the patient fully recovers from the postictal state is status epilepticus. This is a potentially lethal condition if the seizures are generalized tonic-clonic. Death results from systemic complications, such as renal failure with massive myoglobinuria. Hyperthermia, dehydration, cardiac arrhythmias, and other complications of protracted seizure activity may lead to death if the patient is not rapidly and appropriately managed (Table 5-12).

TABLE 5-12.   *Treating Patients with Status Epilepticus*

| |
|---|
| Stabilize autonomic function |
| Check blood gases, glucose, electrolytes, magnesium, calcium |
| Administer thiamine 100 mg IM or IV if alcohol abuse is probable |
| Administer glucose as $D_{50}W$ in a 50-ml bolus IV if hypoglycemia is probable |
| Start intravenous antiepileptic medications |
| Intubate if respiratory effort is depressed |
| Monitor vital signs and cardiac rhythm |
| MR or CT if cause not apparent |
| EEG if diagnosis is in doubt |

## Etiology

The most common cause of status epilepticus in the patient with established epilepsy is poor drug compliance. Patients with no prior history of seizure activity must be investigated for drug or alcohol abuse, meningoencephalitis, subarachnoid hemorrhage, intracranial neoplasia, or other problems that can irritate the cerebral cortex.

## Recognition

Several types of status epilepticus exist. The most easily recognized is the tonic-clonic status. Patients with this type of status exhibit recurrent tonic-clonic seizures and do not return to full consciousness between seizures. Focal motor status or epilepsia partialis continua is manifested by unrelenting focal motor seizure activity, during which the patient has largely normal consciousness. Complex partial or psychomotor status and generalized absence or petit mal status are extremely rare and both produce unremitting alterations in consciousness that are difficult to distinguish from psychoses.

## Treatment

Intravenous antiepileptic medications are essential in the successful management of status epilepticus (Table 5-13). The patient in status should initially be given phenytoin at 50 mg/min up to a total dose of 20 mg/kg/day. Many physicians use diazepam initially in a bolus of 10 or 20 mg IV, but this has the disadvantage of being too readily cleared from the body. Phenytoin is less readily eliminated and therefore provides more protracted protection from recurrent seizure activity. If one IV dose of diazepam administered after the patient has received phenytoin fails to stop the seizures, the diazepam may be repeated every 10 to 20 minutes up to a total dose of 50 mg.

If seizures persist after these measures, the patient may respond to IV phenobarbital given in 260- to 300-mg boluses at 100 mg/min. The IV phenobarbital may be repeated every 15 to 20 minutes until a total dose of 20 mg/kg has been delivered for the day. This total dose should not be administered over less than 1 hour.

As an alternative or as a supplement to phenobarbital, many physicians use IV lorazepam. This may be administered up to a total 1-day dose of 0.1 mg/kg in boluses of 5 to 7 mg.

TABLE 5-13.   *Antiepileptic Medication for Status Epilepticus in Adults*

---
Phenytoin (Dilantin) 20 mg/kg IV at no more than 50 mg/min
Diazepam (Valium) .25 mg/kg IV at no more than 5 mg/min if seizures persist
Repeat diazepam dose every 15 minutes until seizures stop or total dose in 1 day is
 50 mg
Phenobarbital 260 mg IV at no more than 100 mg/min if seizures persist—repeat
 every 20 minutes if seizures persist up to 20 mg/kg/day
Lorazepam 0.1 mg/kg at no more than 2 mg/min IV if seizures persist
Consider general anesthesia if all else fails

---

If all of these measures fail, the patient may require general anesthesia to avoid extensive muscle damage, unremitting hyperthermia, and other consequences of persistent seizure activity. Anesthetics without specific antiepileptic activity will not eliminate the problem, but this intervention will enable the physician to continue investigations that may reveal why the status is so refractory.

## SELECTED REFERENCES

Auer RN, Siesjo BK: Biological differences between ischemia, hypoglycemia, and epilepsy. Ann Neurol *24*:699, 1988.

Delgado-Escueta AV, Treiman DM, Walsh GO: The treatable epilepsies (Part 1). N Engl J Med *308*:1508, 1983.

Farwell JR, Lee YJ, Hirtz DG, et al: Phenobarbital for febrile seizures—Effects on intelligence and on seizure recurrence. N Engl J Med *322*:364, 1990.

Faught E, Peters D, Bartolucci A, et al: Seizures after primary intracerebral hemorrhage. Neurology *39*:1089, 1989.

Freeman JM: Febrile seizures: a consensus on their significance, evaluation, and treatment. Pediatrics *66*:1009, 1980.

Gilman S, Bloedel J, Lechtenberg R: Disorders of the Cerebellum. Philadelphia, F.A. Davis, 1981.

Hopkins A, Garman A, Clarke C: The first seizure in adult life. Lancet *1*:721, 1988.

Lechtenberg R: Epilepsy and the Family. Cambridge, Harvard University Press, 1984.

Lechtenberg R: Seizure Recognition and Treatment. New York, Churchill Livingstone, 1990.

Mattson RH, Cramer JA, Collins JF, et al: Comparison of carbamazepine, phenobarbital, phenytoin, and primidone in partial and secondarily generalized tonic-clonic seizures. N Engl J Med *313*:145, 1985.

Meldrum BS: Pharmacological approaches to the treatment of epilepsy. *In* Meldrum BS, Porter RJ (eds): New Anticonvulsant Drugs. London, John Libbey and Co, 1986.

Murros KE, Evans GW, Toole JF, et al: Cerebral infarction in patients with transient ischemic attacks. J Neurol *236*:182, 1989.

Post RM: Time course of clinical effects of carbamazepine: Implications for mechanism of action. J Clin Psychiatry *49*(4 Suppl):35, 1988.

So N, Gloor P, Quesney F, et al: Depth electrode investigations in patients with bitemporal epileptiform abnormalities. Ann Neurol *25*:423, 1989.

So N, Olivier A, Andermann F, et al: Results of surgical treatment in patients with bitemporal epileptiform abnormalities. Ann Neurol *25*:432, 1989.

Spencer SS: Surgical options for uncontrolled epilepsy. Neurol Clin *4*:669, 1986.

Vining EP, Mellits ED, Dorsen MM, et al: Psychologic and behavioral effects of antiepileptic drugs in children: A double-blind comparison between phenobarbital and valproic acid. Pediatrics *80*:165, 1987.

## Chapter 6
# Speech and Language Disturbances

### APHONIA

Aphonia or mutism is the absence of speech. It may develop with structural brain lesions or psychiatric disorders. Nonstructural causes of mutism not associated with akinetic mutism or psychiatric disease are rare, and when they do occur, they are usually transient. Post-ictal mutism occurs in some patients with epilepsy, and aphonia may be symptomatic of transient ischemic attacks. Obviously, patients with damage to the larynx or associated structures may lose speech, but such local injuries are usually fairly evident.

Aphemia is the inability to combine sounds to produce recognizable speech. The patient may hum or grunt, but more highly structured sounds are extremely difficult for the affected individual. This problem usually arises with lesions in the speech-dominant frontal lobe. That a structural lesion is responsible is usually evident because of associated arm weakness.

Aphonia and aphemia should be investigated with CT or MR imaging of the brain. If no structural problem is apparent and a psychiatric basis for the speech disorder is suspected, an amobarbital interview may establish the integrity of speech mechanisms. This barbiturate will eliminate any voluntary reluctance to speak.

Bilateral thalamic injuries may produce transient aphonia. This was seen more frequently when surgical lesions in the thalami were considered valuable in the treatment of Parkinson disease. The deficit in speech associated with this surgical injury usually resolves over the course of several months.

### APHASIA

Aphasia is a disturbance of language, rather than of the production of speech sounds. The disabilities evidenced with aphasia may include language comprehension, production, repetition, or structuring. Word-finding ability and word recognition may be selectively affected or involved as just one facet of a more complex language disturbance. With some types of aphasia, speech is halting and labored, making it sound nonfluent as well as difficult to understand (Table 6-1). With fluent aphasias, the rhythm and intonation of the individual's speech may sound fairly normal, even if the sounds produced by the patient are nothing more than a meaningless string of phonemes.

Most people control language functions with the left side of the brain. Fewer than 1% of right-handed people are right-hemisphere dominant for speech, and at least 60% of left-handed people are left-hemisphere dominant for speech. Only about 7% of the population is truly left-handed, and so, more than 95% of the general

TABLE 6-1.   *Types of Aphasia*

| Fluent | Nonfluent |
|--------|-----------|
| Receptive (Wernicke's, sensory) | Expressive (Broca's, motor) |
| Conduction | Isolation of speech area |
| Transcortical sensory | Transcortical motor |
| Anomic | Global |

population is left-hemisphere dominant for language. Aphasias usually develop only when the dominant hemisphere is damaged. The most common cause of such damage is stroke. Younger patients recover much more quickly from damage to language areas than do older patients.

**Expressive Aphasia**

The third frontal convolution of the speech-dominant hemisphere is the site usually damaged in patients with a purely expressive, or Broca's, aphasia. A branch occlusion of the middle cerebral artery may produce infarction in this region. With this type of aphasia, speech is halting and labored (Table 6-2). It has a nonfluent, telegraphic quality. Words are often omitted and normal syntax is lost. Comprehension is retained, and the patient is uncomfortably aware of his or her own language errors. Written language is affected in much the same way as is spoken language. The ability to repeat phrases and statements is poor. Reading is impaired.

Neurologic findings usually associated with expressive aphasia include right-facial and right-arm weakness. Visual field cuts do not usually occur with this type of aphasia and right-leg strength may be entirely normal. Using MR scanning and EEG studies, the area of damage can usually be identified and characterized as infarction, hemorrhage, or less commonly, tumor.

**Receptive Aphasia**

Impaired language comprehension is the principal facet of a receptive, or Wernicke's, aphasia. The patient has fluent speech, but cannot follow instructions, repeat phrases, or read. The words produced often contain errors, called paraphasias. Occasionally the

TABLE 6-2.   *Aphasia Characteristics*

| Expressive | Receptive | Global |
|------------|-----------|--------|
| Nonfluent | Fluent | Nonfluent |
| Intact comprehension | Poor comprehension | Poor comprehension |
| Poor repetition | No repetition | No repetition |
| Poor reading | No reading | No reading |
| Poor writing | No writing | No writing |
| Associated facial weakness | Associated field cut | Associated hemiparesis |

patient produces new words, called neologisms, and finds it more difficult to write than to speak. With severe receptive aphasias, the language produced is nonsensical.

Lesions producing receptive aphasias generally involve the posterior third of the superior temporal gyrus. A visual field cut may be associated with temporal lobe damage. Part of the optic radiation from the lateral geniculate, Meyer's loop, swings forward in the temporal lobe before coursing backward to the occipital lobe.

## Conduction Aphasia

The centers for language reception and expression are connected by the arcuate fasciculus, a fiber bundle coursing between the superior temporal gyrus and the inferior frontal lobe. Interruption of this connection produces characteristic language problems, which include pronounced impairment of repetition. Comprehension and expression may be somewhat impaired with conduction aphasia, but they are not as disturbed as is typically seen in receptive or expressive aphasias. The most common site of a lesion producing conduction aphasia is in the dominant parietal lobe. The patient with this aphasia is relatively fluent and has good comprehension of both spoken and written language.

Associated neurologic deficits include a right visual-field cut and right-sided sensory deficit, but the aphasia may occur without any other neurologic signs of disease. Occlusion of a middle cerebral artery branch or a stategically placed tumor may produce this type of aphasia.

## Global Aphasia

Patients with features of both receptive and expressive aphasia have global aphasia. This means that the patient has a nonfluent aphasia with poor comprehension and poor language production. Repetition is virtually impossible and reading as well as writing are lost. Patients with this type of aphasia usually have evidence of extensive dominant-hemisphere damage, with right-arm and face weakness, right-sided sensory deficits, and a right-sided visual field cut also usually evident. Occlusion of a middle cerebral artery is usually responsible for the dominant-hemisphere damage producing this type of deficit. The recovery from global aphasia is usually incomplete, and in many cases does not occur at all.

## Anomic Aphasia

Word-finding difficulty is usually considered a type of aphasia and is called anomic aphasia or anomia. This is a poorly localized problem, which may develop with a variety of focal or diffuse cerebrocortical disturbances ranging from metastatic tumors to progressive degenerative diseases. Anomia and receptive aphasias are problems common early in the evolution of Alzheimer's disease.

## Isolation of the Speech Area

Ischemic damage surrounding but not including the principal speech areas may produce isolation of the speech areas. This type of injury may develop with protracted hypotension, such as that associated with cardiac arrest. Impaired perfusion of watershed areas at the most distal limits of the middle cerebral artery may effectively disconnect Wernicke's area, Broca's area, and the arcuate fasciculus from surrounding cortical structures. The patient manifests this type of injury by exhibiting no spontaneous speech. When he is spoken to, he simply echoes what has been said. This repetition is called echolalia.

## Transcortical Aphasias

In most aphasias, other than isolation of the speech area, repetition is impaired. Exceptions to that rule are the transcortical aphasias. These are poorly localized anatomically but easily recognized clinically. The patient with a transcortical sensory aphasia has excellent repetition despite impaired comprehension. The patient with a transcortical motor aphasia has excellent repetition despite telegraphic spontaneous speech.

## PURE WORD DEAFNESS

Pure word deafness or verbal auditory agnosia is a selective deficit in the comprehension of spoken, but not of written, words. Writing and reading are largely intact, but spoken language is not understood and spontaneous speech is limited if at all present. The patient is aware of the deficit and does not understand his own language production when he tries to speak. This is a rare disorder. It has been described with damage to several different parts of the brain, but it is most commonly associated with lesions connecting the primary auditory area to Wernicke's area.

## DYSLEXIA

Problems with comprehension of written language, dyslexia, may develop in adult life with structural damage to limited areas of the cerebral cortex or may appear idiopathically in childhood. Dyslexia in children is usually unsuspected until the initial efforts to teach the child to read fail repeatedly. Affected children usually have normal speech and writing ability. Reading and writing are routinely affected jointly in adults who develop dyslexia. In adults, dyslexia usually develops as a consequence of damage to the angular gyrus of the dominant parietal lobe. A lesion in this region is presumed to disrupt connections between the visual cortex and Wernicke's area. Associated neurologic deficits include a right-sided visual field cut, a mild right hemiparesis, and agraphia. A lesion in the language-dominant occipital lobe may also produce dyslexia, especially if the corpus callosum is involved, but with preserved writing skills. This is usually called alexia without agraphia.

## DYSARTHRIA

Dysarthria is a disturbance of the clarity, rhythm, or rate of speech. Language structure and meaning are retained with dysarthria, but slurring, slowing, or inappropriate intonation of the patient's speech may make the speech largely unintelligible. Dysarthria may develop with damage to the speech-producing organs, which include the larynx, pharynx, and mouth, or with damage to a variety of nervous system structures. The transient cerebellar dysfunction caused by alcohol intoxication that produces slurring and slowing of speech is indistinguishable from that associated with lithium intoxication or with cerebellar demyelination from multiple sclerosis. All of these neurologic disorders produce dysarthria, but with metabolic disturbances such as alcohol intoxication, the dysarthria is transient, whereas with structural changes such as demyelination or infarction, the dysarthria may be permanent. Patients with cerebellar damage are especially likely to develop a staccato rhythm to their speech, an aberrant speech pattern that is called scanning speech.

## APRAXIA

Apraxia is the inability to perform an action despite the retention of comprehension, coordination, sensation, and strength required. This type of disorder usually occurs in association with expressive aphasia, and it more commonly affects the left arm and leg than the right. Orofacial apraxia, rather than limb apraxia, is the most common of the apraxias. Patients typically cannot perform simple tasks, such as pretending to blow out a match, despite their having no problems with mouth or tongue movements. The lesions underlying these kinds of deficits are presumed to disconnect Broca's area from the motor areas essential for initiating the requested movement.

## SELECTED REFERENCES

Geschwind N: Aphasia. N Engl J Med *284*:654, 1971.
Lechtenberg R, Gilman S: Speech disorders in cerebellar disease. Ann Neurol *3*:285, 1978.
Rowland LP (ed): Merritt's Textbook of Neurology. 8th Ed. Philadelphia, Lea & Febiger, 1989.
Ruff RL, Arbit E: Aphemia resulting from a left frontal hematoma. Neurology *31*:353, 1981.

*Chapter 7*

# Thought and Mood Disorders

Any patient with thought or mood disturbances must be evaluated with attention to the context in which the disturbances arise. The physician must determine whether the changes are acute or chronic, if the setting for the changes involved trauma, febrile illness, intoxication, or a genetic predisposition, and if the apparent defect is static or progressive. Associated neurologic and psychiatric abnormalities must be considered in reaching a diagnosis.

## POST-TRAUMATIC DEMENTIA

Thought or mood disturbances, intellectual impairment, impaired initiative, and poor impulse control may be transient or persistent problems occurring after severe head injury (Table 7-1). If skull fracture, cerebrospinal fluid (CSF) rhinorrhea, or CSF otorrhea develop with the trauma, the injury must be presumed to be severe. Persistent alteration of consciousness, seizures at the time of impact or subsequently, and persistent cranial nerve dysfunctions are additional indications of severe head trauma.

### Cerebral Concussion and Contusion

After sustaining massive head trauma, the patient may exhibit transient or persistent cognitive problems. If thinking is clouded only briefly and no structural damage is evident in the brain, the injury is considered a concussion. If the brain has focal damage with bleeding or edema caused by the blow to the head, the injury is considered a contusion (Fig. 7-1). The contusion is a more serious injury, because it is more likely to produce persistent cognitive problems and may even serve as the focus for a seizure disorder.

### Acute Subdural and Epidural Hematomas

If head trauma is sufficiently massive or strategically placed, the patient may hemorrhage into the subdural or epidural space. Epidural bleeding requires that a high-pressure artery be breached, because the epidural space in the cranial vault is a potential space between the dura mater and the periosteum of the skull. Laceration of the middle meningeal artery is the most common cause of epidural hematomas. Acute subdural hematomas may develop with a blow involving considerably less force than that required to produce an epidural hematoma. Very young children may develop subdural hematomas after vigorous shaking, and elderly people may develop them after relatively slight head trauma. Consciousness, as well as clarity of thinking, is usually impaired as either the subdural or

TABLE 7-1.  *Causes of Memory Impairment*

| Transient | Permanent |
|---|---|
| Head trauma | Head trauma |
| Alcoholic blackouts | Wernicke's encephalopathy |
| Meningoencephalitis | Encephalitis |
| Cerebral arteritis | Cerebral neoplasms |
| Transient ischemic attacks | Cerebral infarction |
| Complicated migraine | Neurosyphilis |
| Sepsis | Severe hypoglycemia |
| Electroconvulsive therapy | Protracted anoxia |
| Meningeal carcinomatosis | Subarachnoid hemorrhage |
| Basilar impression | Normal pressure hydrocephalus |
| Mild hypoglycemia | |
| Metabolic encephalopathy | |
| Seizures | |
| Fugue states | |

epidural hematoma expands. The epidural hematoma usually expands much more rapidly than the subdural and is much more immediately life-threatening. With either lesion, patients die from herniation of the brain.

### Focal Brain Damage

With penetrating injuries of the skull, focal deficits are likely because of damage to the underlying cerebral cortex; but even without skull fracture or penetration, extensive brain damage may occur with blunt injuries. The most common setting for focal brain damage

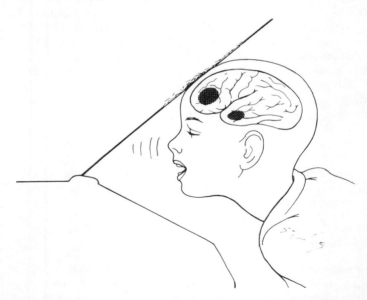

FIG. 7-1. In motor vehicle accidents, the frontal poles of the frontal and temporal lobes may be contused and produce dementia. (With permission from Lechtenberg R: Epilepsy and the Family. Cambridge, Harvard University Press, 1984.)

with trauma is motor vehicle accidents. The frontal and temporal lobes are most often involved. With deceleration injuries, the sort that occur when an individual hits the windshield of a car face first, the frontal and temporal poles may suffer contusions or massive hematoma formation intracerebrally. Damage to the frontal lobe may affect mood changes substantially, making the patient less animated and independent. Damage to the temporal lobe may compromise memory or, if the damage is extensive enough on the dominant side, produce a receptive aphasia. If the head is struck with a blunt object, such as a metal pipe, the brain may be contused at both the site of impact and at the site opposite the impact. This type of contre-coûp injury develops from acceleration of the brain caused by the impact with compression of cerebral tissue occurring against the opposite side of the skull.

### Subarachnoid Hemorrhage

Hemorrhage into the subarachnoid space may occur spontaneously, from aneurysms, from arteriovenous malformations, or from head trauma. The blood causes cognitive dysfunction in most individuals and impaired consciousness in many. Blood is irritating to the lining of the subarachnoid space and may produce a chemical meningitis as well as focal spasms along the cerebral blood vessels.

## AMNESIA

Impaired recall develops in many neurologic conditions. Head trauma may produce transient or permanent memory disorders, but the type of identity loss associated with a blow to the head that is depicted in many fictional works is pure fiction itself. Head trauma sufficient to produce disorientation will not spare other short-term and long-term aspects of recall. Transient global amnesia, in which the ability to recall old memories and to lay down new memories is disrupted for minutes or hours, is presumed to occur with transient ischemia to the temporal lobes. Persistence of this type of memory disturbance is rare. Individuals are presumed to be susceptible to this type of cognitive disorder if they have preexisting damage in the contralateral temporal lobe. Bilateral temporal lobe strokes, especially those involving the hippocampus, may produce severe and persistent memory disturbances. Unilateral hippocampal damage may cause problems with learning and memory if the dominant hemisphere is the one affected.

### Confabulation

Some individuals with profound memory loss may deny any problems with memory and glibly confabulate events in the recent and remote past. This occurs most commonly in the Wernicke-Korsakoff syndrome, a metabolic disorder of brain function associated with thiamine deficiency. The cognitive disorder is classically referred to as a Korsakoff psychosis. Periaqueductal and hypothalamic hemorrhagic necrosis are the structural changes evident with the most rapidly progressive form of this syndrome.

## Postictal Confusion

Transient thought disorders routinely occur after generalized tonic-clonic, complex partial, and other types of seizures. This postictal confusion may consist of disorientation, delusions, amnesia, aphasia, or other more complex cognitive disorders. The postictal problems usually last only a few minutes, but some patients remain impaired for hours, days, or, much more rarely, weeks. Seizures do not cause progressive cognitive impairment: the postictal confusion invariably clears entirely.

## INFECTIOUS DISEASES

Infectious diseases causing meningitis, encephalitis, or meningoencephalitis may produce severe thought disorders. The damage done by the infection may be transient or permanent, the type of organism in large part determining the probability of permanent damage. The responsible organisms range from parasites to viruses (Fig. 7-2). The long-term sequelae of the infections or infestations range from epilepsy to focal weakness. The short-term problems usually include cognitive impairment.

### Bacterial Meningoencephalitis

The bacteria affecting newborns are most often Escherichia coli or sexually transmitted organisms, such as Treponema pallidum. Congenital or intrauterine infections with toxoplasmosis and syphilis may produce severe retardation, as well as developmental disabil-

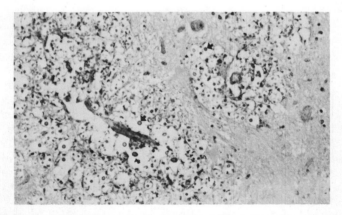

FIG. 7-2. A wide variety of organisms may produce dementia. This photomicrograph reveals perivascular infiltrates of cryptococci in an immunodeficient patient with dementia. (With permission from Lechtenberg R: Seizure Recognition and Treatment. New York, Churchill Livingstone, 1990.)

ities. Infants and young children with meningitis or meningoencephalitis usually have Hemophilus influenzae as the responsible
agent. Young adults are especially vulnerable to H. influenzae and
meningococcal infections. Older adults most often develop pneumococcal meningitis. Individuals at any age may have tuberculous
meningitis. Immunosuppressed individuals, such as those with AIDS,
are especially vulnerable to rapidly progressive neurosyphilis. Renal
transplant recipients receiving immunosuppressive agents have special susceptibility to Listeria monocytogenes, an organism that may
produce focal encephalitis, generalized meningitis, or brain abscesses.

### Neurosyphilis

Tertiary syphilis was a leading cause of progressive dementia
before the advent of penicillin. General paresis, a degenerative brain
disease characterized by direct invasion of the brain parenchyma
by the spirochete Treponema pallidum produced memory and thought
disturbances that often involved delusions and confabulations. With
the spread of AIDS, neurosyphilis is resurging. Primary syphilis is
evolving into tertiary syphilis over the course of weeks, rather than
years, in patients with AIDS. The dementia of neurosyphilis in these
patients may be masked by the progressive dementia caused by HIV
infection of the brain.

### Viral Encephalitis

Several viruses produce dementia over the course of weeks, months,
or years. The virus may do its damage prenatally, as well as during
infancy, childhood, or adult life. Intrauterine rubella infections may
lead to autism in the infant, as well as to deafness and other neurologic disabilities. Cytomegalovirus is also a major cause of intrauterine brain damage, often associated with congenital calcification
of the basal ganglia and retardation. Less common viral agents, such
as eastern and western equine encephalitis, may produce childhood
disease with speech and cognitive problems that may become more
obvious as the child matures.

**Herpes Simplex.**   Cognitive and affective changes usually occur
early in the evolution of herpetic encephalitis. Disturbances of memory and mood are often prominent, with irritability sometimes pre-
ceding obvious encephalopathy by days or weeks. Seizures may be
the first manifestation of encephalitis. Patients with normal im-
munity usually have a fulminant, necrotizing encephalitis. Type 2
virus usually causes disease during the neonatal period, after which,
type 1 is the more likely strain to produce disease. In patients with
AIDS, either type 2 or type 1 may become established in the brain
and produce an atypically diffuse and nonhemorrhagic encephalitis.

CT or MR scanning of the affected individual usually reveals
prominent, unilateral temporal lobe edema and focal breakdown of
the blood-brain barrier. The EEG may exhibit periodic slow or
sharp wave discharges, most prominently in the temporal lobe leads.
Changes in the cerebrospinal fluid are usually limited to a slight

increase in the white blood cell count and protein content. A few red blood cells may also appear in the CSF. Management of affected patients with vidarabine and other antiviral drugs has resulted in less mortality than is customarily seen without intervention.

**Subacute Sclerosing Panencephalitis (SSPE).** SSPE is a rare, relatively late sequela of measles or, much less commonly, mumps infection. Children or young adults with this disorder exhibit a dementia that appears months to years after the original viral exanthema and evolves over the course of months. Patients usually develop myoclonic jerks as the disease progresses. The EEG may show a periodic discharge. Computed tomography of the brain is generally unrevealing. The damage incurred with this disease is lethal.

**Progressive Multifocal Leukoencephalopathy.** In a variety of disorders of immune function, patients may develop demyelination associated with a papovavirus infection. Because this demyelination usually involves multiple areas of the cerebral white matter, the disorder is called progressive multifocal leukoencephalopathy (PML). Dementia is a common presenting sign with this disease, but focal weakness, personality changes, and aphasias are also likely. The JC, BK, and SV 40 strains of papovavirus are the ones usually responsible for the demyelination. Currently, this disease most often appears in patients with AIDS, but it was initially described in patients with Hodgkin's disease, other lymphomas, lymphocytic leukemias, and sarcoid.

Characteristic of the lesions developing with this viral disease is scattered demyelination with little or no associated inflammation. The oligodendroglial cells have large nuclei with viral inclusion bodies, and astrocytes may be enlarged and multinucleated. The diagnosis is usually based on CT or MR findings of multifocal demyelination in the appropriate setting.

Death ensues within a few months if the disease is untreated. Antiviral therapies have produced remissions in some patients.

**Kuru.** Kuru is a lethal neurodegenerative disorder that produces both affective and cognitive disorders early in its evolution. Tremors and ataxia develop as cerebellar damage evolves. It is caused by a virus that appears to be transmitted primarily through direct contact with infected nervous system tissue. The course of the disease extends over years, with the final phase of deterioration lasting 3 to 9 months. Because so protracted a course was considered extraordinary for a progressive viral illness, kuru was called a slow virus when it was first described among the Fore Islanders of New Guinea.

The virus is related to the causative agent in Creutzfeldt-Jakob disease. Both produce a characteristic spongiform encephalopathy. Neither evokes a substantial inflammatory response in the brain. Both are invariably fatal.

**Creutzfeldt-Jakob Disease.** Creutzfeldt-Jakob disease is a slow viral disease that causes progressive dementia and death. Unlike kuru, which is limited to isolated enclaves in New Guinea, it occurs in densely populated areas of the United States. About one person in a million develops symptoms of the disease. These include global intellectual deterioration, lethargy, weight loss, irritability, myoclonic jerks, clumsiness, tremors, visual loss, and paranoia. The illness progresses over the course of a few to several months before the patient dies. Terminally, patients develop akinetic mutism.

Diagnostic studies short of brain biopsy to identify the spongiform encephalopathy include CSF and EEG evaluations. The CSF has an elevated level of protein without other signs of inflammation. The EEG often reveals irregular bursts of high-amplitude slow waves or regularly recurring spikes or sharp waves at 1-second intervals (Fig. 7-3). The 1-per-second discharges are occasionally polyspike discharges. MR or CT scanning reveals generalized atrophy late in the course of the illness.

Biopsy of the brains of these patients reveals plaques in the cerebellum that react with periodic acid Schiff stain (PAS). Fluid accumulations in dendritic and astrocytic processes are evident and give the brain its characteristic spongiform appearance. Damage to the basal ganglia is usually prominent.

**AIDS Encephalopathy.**   An increasingly common cause of dementia is infection with the human immunodeficiency viruses (HIVs). The most common strain in industrialized nations is HIV-1, but both HIV-1 and HIV-2 have been associated with a progressive dementing illness. These viruses cause the acquired immune deficiency syndrome (AIDS) and therefore may produce dementia by allowing opportunistic infections to evolve in the brain, but the HIVs themselves produce progressive encephalopathy, with global intellectual deterioration evolving as the disease becomes more fulminant. The viruses responsible have been well-characterized: they are RNA retroviruses that infect macrophages and other elements of the immune system. It is by way of macrophages that the virus appears to gain access to the brain and spinal cord.

Zidovudine (AZT) and dideoxyinosine (ddI), currently used to suppress AIDS, may be helpful in limiting the evolution of AIDS

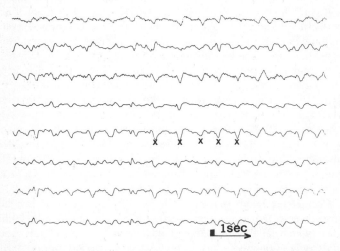

FIG. 7-3. Periodic slow waves, such as those occurring on this EEG at 1 Hz (x), may occur with Creutzfeldt-Jakob disease. (With permission from Lechtenberg R: Epilepsy and the Family. Cambridge, Harvard University Press, 1984.)

encephalopathy, but experience with these antiviral agents and with AIDS encephalopathy itself has been too limited to assume that the drugs can effectively treat the encephalopathy.

## VASCULAR DISEASE

Vascular disease is a common cause of focal or diffuse cerebro-cortical dysfunction. Vessel occlusion from atheromatous plaques in arterial walls or endothelial hyperplasia accounts for much of the disease seen in industrialized nations. Inflammatory disease of blood vessels is common in regions with high levels of meningovascular diseases, such as meningovascular syphilis. Hemorrhages may develop without apparent vascular disease if the patient has thrombocytopenia, hemophilia, or other causes of coagulopathy. Hemorrhages develop much more commonly in patients with chronic hypertension, aneurysms, or arteriovenous malformations.

### Stroke

Strokes are structural injuries to the brain or spinal cord caused by ischemia or hemorrhage. Neurologic damage occurs with these vascular accidents by way of several mechanisms, including direct tissue compression with massive intracerebral hemorrhage and hypoxic damage with vascular occlusions. A variety of chronic illnesses and activities increase the risk of stroke. In the United States, risk factors for the development of stroke include chronic hypertension, heart disease, cigarette smoking, diabetes mellitus, and hyperlipidemia. Strokes may occur with emboli originating in the heart or elsewhere, but emboli are the sole cause of infarction in only about 1 of 12 patients with ischemic brain injuries.

Severe strokes may cause substantial weakness, numbness, or loss of coordination without substantially affecting intellectual ability. This is especially true if memory and language are undisturbed by the cerebrovascular accident. Lacunar strokes, millimeter-sized infarctions often associated with hypertensive vascular disease, typically do not cause intellectual disturbances unless small-vessel disease is so widespread that a multi-infarct dementia develops. Men are at greater risk for multi-infarct dementia than are women. The appearance of dementia is more directly related to the site of the ischemic injury than to the total volume of brain tissue damage. Specific cognitive problems that usually arise from strokes injuring strategic areas of the brain include the Gerstmann syndrome and a variety of neglect syndromes.

**Gerstmann Syndrome.**    Damage to the dominant parietal hemisphere may cause a collection of distinctive cognitive problems called the Gerstmann syndrome. Major elements of the syndrome include (1) right-left confusion; (2) finger agnosia, the inability to identify fingers by name; (3) dyscalculia, problems with calculations; and (4) agraphia, impaired writing. With damage to either parietal lobe, patients also exhibit constructional apraxia, an impairment of drawing, and visual field defects, a consequence of damage to the subcortical optic radiation. Conduction aphasias or other language problems appear along with the Gerstmann syndrome in many patients. Specific tests usually reveal problems with word finding and maze learning.

**Denial of Illness.** With nondominant parietal lobe damage, patients may exhibit anosognosia, the denial of disability. The hemiplegic side is described as normal by the affected patient. If the paralyzed limb is placed in the patient's field of vision, he may even deny that the immobile limb belongs to him. When asked to perform an activity with the paralyzed limb, the patient may claim that he did what was asked even though no movement of the limb occurred. Even more peculiar is the patient who provides complex explanations for why the paralyzed limbs should not be moved and who insists that no fundamental problem exists with the hemiplegic side.

## Systemic Lupus Erythematosus (SLE)

SLE may produce transient neurologic deficits in association with focal inflammatory disease. The most common central nervous system problems developing with lupus are seizures and psychosis. These are often sensitive to corticosteroid treatment.

## METABOLIC DISEASES

Patients with kidney or liver disease may develop encephalopathy as their organ failure progresses. Stupor, disorientation, and memory problems are common with these metabolic encephalopathies, but some patients have florid hallucinations and paranoid delusions. Thought and mood disorders also develop with thyroid disease, adrenal insufficiency, parathyroid dysfunction, and Cushing disease, but these cognitive and affective disorders are more readily linked to hormonal disorders than to strictly metabolic problems. Glucose and calcium disturbances are especially common bases for thought and mood disturbances. Hypoxia, such as that associated with a pulmonary embolus, is also a common basis for cognitive disturbances.

Arsenic, lead, manganese, mercury, and thallium at nonlethal doses may disturb memory. Other signs of poisoning, such as hair loss and peripheral neuropathy with thallium, tremor and affective disorders with mercury, or wrist drop and lethargy with lead, usually suggest the metabolic basis for the progressive cognitive disorder. Much of the disability produced by these poisons is reversible (Table 7-2). This is not true of the dementia caused by carbon monoxide poisoning.

Vitamin deficiency and other forms of malnutrition produce transient or persistent dementia, depending on the severity of the deprivation and the age of the individual when the deficiency was suffered. Nicotinic acid deficiency produced pellagra with its characteristic dementia and dermatitis. Thiamine deficiency may lead to Wernicke's encephalopathy, as well as the systemic problems of beriberi.

TABLE 7-2. *Dementia*

| Treatable Causes | Untreatable Causes |
|---|---|
| Depression | Alzheimer's disease |
| Recurrent seizures | Progressive supranuclear palsy |
| Intoxication | Carbon monoxide poisoning |
| Poisoning | Protracted hypoxia |
| Benign brain tumors | Cerebral infarction |
| Chronic subdural hematomas | Malignant brain tumor |
| Brain abscess | Creutzfeldt-Jakob disease |
| Electrolyte disturbances | Kuru |
| Uremia | Most viral meningoencephalitides |
| Hepatic encephalopathy | |
| Pellagra | |
| Systemic lupus erythematosus | |
| Combined systems disease | |
| Endocrine disturbances | |
| Progressive multifocal leukoencephalopathy | |
| Bacterial meningoencephalitis | |

Substance abuse is an exceedingly common cause of cognitive disorders. Alcoholism, even with adequate dietary thiamine, probably induces some memory impairment after years of ethanol abuse. Other addictive drugs produce a more transient disturbance in memory or judgment. Cocaine use gives the new user a feeling of competence in a variety of physical and intellectual activities, but the feeling of competence is not accompanied by an objective improvement in performance. With persistent use, judgment and cognitive performance deteriorate as addiction develops. Marijuana-smoking has been associated with short-term problems with memory.

## DEGENERATIVE DISEASES OF THE BRAIN

### Alzheimer's Disease

Alzheimer's disease is the most common degenerative disease of the central nervous system. It produces a slowly progressive dementia, often characterized by receptive language difficulties, progressive memory impairment, paranoid ideation, and psychomotor slowing.

Pathologic features in the brain include neurofibrillary tangles, senile plaques, and neuronal dropout. The neurofibrils are intracellular elements of dendrites and axons that are essential for intracellular transport of materials. Tangles of these structures probably denote severe metabolic dysfunction within individual neurons. Senile plaques are regions in the brain where degenerating nerve processes have accumulated around an amyloid core. Neuronal loss occurs predominantly in association areas of the cortex, those areas in which different neurologic activities are integrated. The extent of pathologic change correlates roughly with the severity of dementia exhibited by the patient. No inflammatory infiltrate occurs with these plaques. The amyloid material in the plaque has been characterized as a beta-pleated sheet of protein similar to the short-chain elements of immunoglobulin molecules. Brain volume and weight decrease as the disease progresses, and the brain assumes a characteristically atrophic appearance.

Identical pathologic features occur with other diseases, such as Down syndrome, progressive supranuclear palsy, Parkinson disease, and postencephalitic parkinsonism, but the association of these pathologic changes with the characteristic neurologic signs and symptoms of Alzheimer's disease establishes the diagnosis. MR or CT studies of the brain usually reveal cerebral atrophy and hydrocephalus ex vacuo, the compensatory enlargement of the ventricles that occurs with cerebral atrophy, fairly early in the evolution of signs and symptoms. The EEG of affected individuals shows slowing of the background rhythm into the theta frequency ranges of 4 to 7 Hz. If the disease occurs before the age of 60, brain biopsy may be necessary to exclude treatable causes of dementia.

The cause of Alzheimer's disease is still unknown, but most investigators favor a metabolic or viral etiology. No treatment has substantially affected the course of the disease. The dementia usually progresses inexorably for a few years until death intervenes. Patients generally die from infection, malnutrition, or trauma.

## Pick's Disease

Pick's disease is a relatively uncommon cause of dementia that produces clinical signs and symptoms largely indistinguishable from Alzheimer's disease. The cortical atrophy occurring with this disease is primarily in the frontal and temporal lobes. The memory disturbance often spares recent memory early in the evolution of the disease. Many patients exhibit inclusions, called Pick bodies, in neurons when these are exposed to silver stains. Neuronal loss is usually substantial in the most atrophic parts of the brain. This is an untreatable disease that shortens life expectancy to the same extent as does Alzheimer's disease.

## Parkinson Disease

Parkinson disease (see Chapter 9) is usually considered a movement disorder rather than a dementing illness, but dementia may be the initial manifestation of Parkinson disease. Although it is rarely the first symptom, dementia becomes apparent in more than half the affected individuals as their disease progresses. Memory formation, orientation, and construction, rather than language ability and recall of remote information, are primarily affected. The receptive aphasia commonly observed with Alzheimer's disease does not usually appear. Treatments for the movement disorder of Parkinson disease do not substantially affect the progression of dementia occurring with this disease.

## Huntington Disease

Huntington disease, like Parkinson disease, is a movement disorder that has dementia as a prominent component (see Chapter

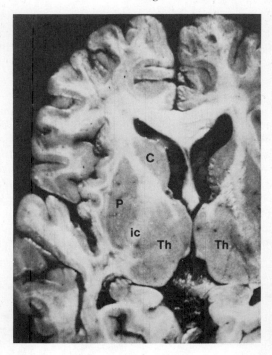

FIG. 7-4. In Huntington disease, the caudate nucleus (C) usually exhibits obvious atrophy even before dementia is substantial (P = putamen, ic = internal capsule, Th = thalamus).

9). Rather than memory disturbances, the first evidence of dementia in Huntington disease is usually a personality change with prominent irritability, impaired judgment, and poor insight. Some individuals become apathetic and indecisive. The thought and mood disorders may progress even if chorea does not appear as the disease evolves. Evidence of caudate atrophy on MR or CT scan may be diagnostic (Fig. 7-4).

### Progressive Supranuclear Palsy (Steele-Richardson-Olszewski Syndrome)

Progressive supranuclear palsy causes dementia associated with parkinsonism. It is much less common than Parkinson disease; patients with this syndrome exhibit gait and memory problems, as well as irritability and suspiciousness. As the disease evolves, affected individuals develop ophthalmoplegia, slurred speech, and dystonic posturing. Unlike patients with Parkinson disease, tremors in patients with this syndrome are usually subtle or absent. The ophthalmoplegia starts with impaired downward gaze. Saccadic eye movements slow as the patient deteriorates, but reflex stimulation of the brainstem nuclei controlling eye movements reveals that the impairment is above the level of the ocular motor nuclei.

The disease evolves over the course of years. Death intervenes within 4 to 7 years in the majority of affected individuals. Death results from infection, dehydration, malnutrition, or trauma.

## HYDROCEPHALUS

Any obstruction to the flow or resorption of cerebrospinal fluid may produce focal or generalized hydrocephalus (Fig. 7-5). If the communication between the ventricles and the subarachnoid space overlying the spinal cord is blocked, the hydrocephalus is considered obstructive. If no such block exists, it is a nonobstructive hydrocephalus. Either obstructive or nonobstructive hydrocephalus is usually associated with dementia or retardation if it persists.

Hydrocephalus may appear at any age. It often develops in utero with infections that obliterate the aqueduct of Sylvius or induce developmental abnormalities in the foramina of Luschka and Ma-

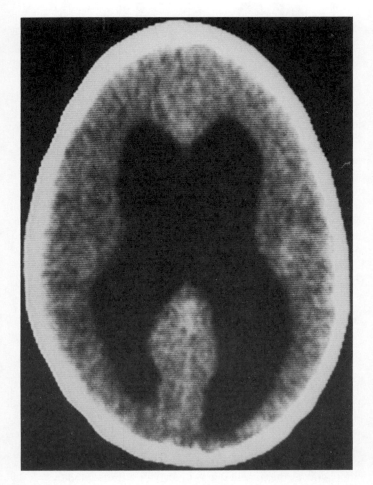

FIG. 7-5. Massive enlargement of the lateral ventricles, as seen on this CT scan, is usually associated with dementia.

gendie. Irritative lesions later in life, such as those associated with subarachnoid hemorrhage or meningitis, may produce hydrocephalus, presumably by interfering with the absorption of cerebrospinal fluid. Third ventricular masses and tumors obstructing the aqueduct of Sylvius or the fourth ventricle may produce hydrocephalus with enlargement of only part of the ventricular system. Brain tumors in children often cause severe hydrocephalus because they obstruct CSF flow through the posterior fossa. Cerebellar tumors, such as medulloblastomas and astrocytomas, and ependymal tumors are common causes of hydrocephalus developing in early childhood.

### Hydrocephalus Ex Vacuo

Hydrocephalus ex vacuo, strictly speaking, is not a true hydrocephalus. It is enlargement of the ventricles that occurs over the entire ventricular system or over a segment of that system as a response to local collapse of brain tissue. It appears with generalized atrophy during the evolution of Alzheimer's disease or with encephalomalacia after cerebral infarction.

### Normal Pressure Hydrocephalus (NPH)

Patients with progressive dementia, gait difficulty, and urinary incontinence occasionally exhibit a nonobstructive hydrocephalus with normal CSF pressure. If this is a true hydrocephalus, rather than a hydrocephalus ex vacuo, it is considered a syndrome that may respond to ventriculoperitoneal shunt placement. The patient with this syndrome usually deteriorates over the course of months or years. Signs and symptoms generally develop at an earlier age than characteristically seen with Alzheimer's disease. Most affected individuals develop problems with gait or memory in their fifth decade of life. Although recovery may be substantial with shunting, many patients exhibit recurrent deterioration after transient improvement.

For many years, the diagnosis of normal pressure hydrocephalus was confirmed by introducing a radionuclide into the CSF and following its pattern of distribution in and elimination from the ventricular system. The typical patient with normal pressure hydrocephalus exhibited intraventricular stasis of the radionuclide and delayed elimination from the CSF. Because shunting may help patients who do not have the typical pattern of radionuclide handling and because many patients with the typical pattern have other causes of dementia apparent at autopsy, many physicians recommend proceeding with the minimally traumatic shunting procedure if the patient has the typical signs and symptoms of NPH.

## ENDOCRINE DISORDERS

Severe hypothyroidism may produce psychomotor slowing, flat affect, impaired memory, inattention, and depression. This is sometimes called myxedema madness. In addition to cognitive and affective disorders, these patients often exhibit ataxia, carpal tunnel syndrome, weakness, and hearing loss. Gradual replacement of the deficient thyroid hormone will correct all of the neurologic problems.

Severe dementia without agitation occasionally develops with hyperthyroidism in the elderly. This is called apathetic hyperthyroidism and responds to reduction of thyroid activity. Similarly, the cognitive dysfunction associated with adrenal and parathyroid dysfunction may be corrected with management of the hormonal disturbance.

## SELECTED REFERENCES

Anlar B, Yalaz K, Ustacelebi S: Symptoms, signs and laboratory data in 80 cases of subacute sclerosing panencephalitis. Rev Neurol *144*:829, 1988.

Brown HR, Goller NL, Rudelli RD, et al: Postmortem detection of measles virus in non-neural tissues in subacute sclerosing panencephalitis. Ann Neurol *26*:263, 1989.

Casmiro M, D'Alessandro R, Cacciatore FM, et al: Risk factors for the syndrome of ventricular enlargement with gait apraxia (idiopathic normal pressure hydrocephalus): A case-control study. J Neurol Neurosurg Psychiatry *52*:847, 1989.

Englund E, Brun A, Alling C: White matter changes in dementia of Alzheimer's type. Biochemical and neuropathological correlates. Brain *111*:1425, 1988.

Gibson RM, Stephenson GC: Aggressive management of severe closed head trauma: Time for reappraisal. Lancet *2*:369, 1989.

Girotti F, Soliveri P, Carella F, et al: Dementia and cognitive impairment in Parkinson's disease. J Neurol Neurosurg Psychiatry *51*:1498, 1988.

Guidotti M, Anzalone N, Morabito A, Landi G: A case-control study of transient global amnesia. Neurol Neurosurg Psychiatry *52*:320, 1989.

Knopman DS, Christensen KJ, Schut LJ, et al: The spectrum of imaging and neuropsychological findings in Pick's disease. Neurology *39*:326, 1989.

Lechtenberg R: Seizure Recognition and Treatment. New York, Churchill Livingstone, 1990.

Lechtenberg R: AIDS in the Nervous System. New York, Churchill Livingstone, 1989.

Lechtenberg R: The Psychiatrist's Guide to Diseases of the Nervous System. New York, John Wiley, 1982.

Lukehart SA, Hook EW III, Baker-Zander SA, et al: Invasion of the central nervous system by Treponema pallidum: Implications for diagnosis and treatment. Ann Intern Med *109*:855, 1988.

Meyer JS, McClinic KL, Rogers RL, et al: Aetiological considerations and risk factors for multi-infarct dementia. J Neurol Neurosurg Psychiatry *51*:1489, 1988.

Rinne JO, Rummukainen J, Paljarvi L, Rinne UK: Dementia in Parkinson's disease is related to neuronal loss in the medial substantia nigra. Ann Neurol *26*:47, 1989.

Roberts GW: Immunocytochemistry of neurofibrillary tangles in dementia pugilistica and Alzheimer's disease: Evidence for common genesis. Lancet *2*:8626, 1988.

von Cramon DY, Hebel N, Schuri U: Verbal memory and learning in unilateral posterior cerebral infarction: A report on 30 cases. Brain *111*:1061, 1988.

Wolters EC, Hische EAH, Tutuarima JA, et al: Central nervous system involvement in early and late syphilis: The problem of asymptomatic neurosyphilis. J Neurol Sci *88*:229, 1988.

*Chapter 8*

# Sexual and Urogenital Problems

Most sexual problems are either psychologic, urologic, or neurologic. Urologic problems may be from local disease or neurologic dysfunction. Either may arise from damage to the peripheral or central nervous system. Problems with sexual and urologic function often occur together because many of the neurologic structures essential for sexual function are also essential for bladder control.

## DISTURBED AROUSAL AND ORGASM

Problems with orgasm in men are usually associated with impotence, the inability to achieve or sustain penile erection. Women actually have impaired orgasm more commonly than do men, but their anorgasmia is less frequently reported or investigated. Impotence unassociated with obvious neurologic or urologic disease occurs in about 7% of men. Anorgasmia during sexual intercourse is reported by as many as 1 in 3 otherwise healthy women. Chronic pain routinely impairs sexual interest and activity.

## IMPOTENCE

Impotence may develop because of vascular, neurologic, or simply structural penile problems. Common diseases such as diabetes mellitus and chronic alcoholism produce sexual problems, including impotence, through a variety of mechanisms. Illicit and prescription drugs also account for many cases of impotence (Table 8-1). Antihypertensive agents are especially likely to impair potency. Certain antiepileptics, such as phenobarbital and primidone, frequently produce impotence in the men taking them, but most antiepileptics, including phenytoin and carbamazepine, impair sexual performance in only rare individuals.

One largely structural cause of impotence is Peyronie syndrome, a disorder in which a plaque of fibrous tissue forms in and around the corpora cavernosa and spongiosum. This fibrous band results from idiopathic inflammatory disease. During erection, the penis is deformed, with its most distal component remaining flaccid.

Damage to the lumbosacral spinal cord may in turn damage reflex centers essential for normal erection. Damage to the cauda equina routinely produces impaired gait, impotence, and urinary incontinence in affected men, a combination of problems called the cauda equina syndrome.

### Iatrogenic Hyposexuality

Many drugs cause sexual dysfunction in both men and women. Antiepileptic medications may cause anorgasmia as well as impo-

TABLE 8-1. *Drugs Affecting Sexual Function*

| Depressing Libido | Causing Impotence |
| --- | --- |
| Alcohol | Methyldopa |
| Marijuana | Guanethidine |
| Barbiturates | Clonidine |
| Acetazolamide | Propranolol |
| Cocaine | Phenobarbital |
| Diazepam | Chlorothiazide |
| Digoxin | Hydrochlorothiazide |
| Doxepin | Spironolactone |
| Heroin | Reserpine |
| Imipramine | Phenothiazines |
| Methyldopa | Imipramine |
| Propranolol | Alcohol |
| Spironolactone | Primidone |
| Bromide salts | |

tence. Pelvic surgery or irradiation or genital surgery may produce sexual dysfunction. After prostatectomy, men may be unable to achieve erections, but this is a relatively uncommon result of the surgery especially if it is performed transurethrally.

## Spinal Cord Disease

Genital function persists even after complete transection of the spinal cord if the reflex centers in the lumbosacral spinal cord are preserved. Damage to lumbar or sacral segments may interfere with erection and ejaculation in men or with lubrication and penile accommodation in women. Problems with genital function may lead to dyspareunia, pain on intercourse, in either men or women.

Myelodysplasia, the disturbance of spinal cord development, may cause substantial sexual dysfunction, but associated neurologic deficits, such as bladder and bowel dysfunction and paraparesis, usually suggest the underlying defect. Syringomyelia, a cyst in the spinal cord, may cause sexual problems even if the cyst forms primarily above lumbosacral segments of the spinal cord. It causes problems by disturbing long tracts to areas controlling sexual reflexes. Other primarily long-tract diseases of the spinal cord include multiple sclerosis and tabes dorsalis. Tabes dorsalis produces damage in the posterior columns and dorsal spinal roots; it is one of many manifestations of neurosyphilis. With the spread of the acquired immunodeficiency syndrome (AIDS), neurosyphilis is becoming more common.

## Diabetes Mellitus

Impotence occurs in about 60% of men with diabetes mellitus. Neuropathy and vascular disease both contribute to the sexual dysfunction. The neuropathy affects the pudendal nerve, the principal source of strictly neural control of genital reactions. Both sympathetic and parasympathetic components of the autonomic nervous system are essential for normal sexual function in men and women, and diabetes damages both of these components.

## Brain Damage

Acutely after a massive stroke, patients often exhibit urinary incontinence. Even if the patient has dense hemiplegia as a result of the stroke, bladder and sexual function will usually return over the course of months or years. Individuals with more generalized brain damage, such as boxers, may have an irreversible loss of sexual function.

## Shy-Drager Syndrome

Impotence is the most common initial complaint in men who develop Shy-Drager syndrome, a progressive disturbance of the autonomic nervous system that eventually produces parkinsonism. Men with Parkinson disease also may develop impotence as their degenerative disease progresses, but in Shy-Drager syndrome, the dysautonomia is an early and evident sign of neurologic disease.

## Endocrine Disorders

Sexual dysfunction may develop with endocrine disturbances during maturation; but more commonly, problems with hormonal regulation produce problems for adults. Hyperprolactinemia associated with pituitary tumors impairs libido in both sexes and may produce impotence in men. Hyperthyroidism may depress testosterone levels.

## DYSPAREUNIA

Dyspareunia is pain on intercourse. It is a common complaint in women after the climacteric because of thinning of the vulvar and vaginal epithelia and diminution in vaginal secretions. With cervical or uterine cancer, women may complain of dyspareunia late in the progression of disease. Superficial lesions on the genitalia may also produce pain, depending on the character of the problem causing the lesion. Herpetic ulcers may produce burning pain on attempted intercourse, whereas syphilitic chancres are insensitive and do not cause dyspareunia. Spasms of the musculature of the outer third of the vagina, a condition usually called vaginismus, may cause pain on attempted intercourse for both the man and the woman. Men experience dyspareunia if erection is incomplete, such as occurs with Peyronie syndrome.

## HYPERSEXUALITY

Excessive sexual activity occurs with rare syndromes triggered by brain damage. The persistence of sexual behavior in inappropriate contexts makes the observed sexuality abnormal.

## Kleine-Levin Syndrome

Hypersexuality associated with hypersomnia and hyperphagia in adolescent men is called the Kleine-Levin syndrome. The cause of this disorder is unknown. It is usually self-limited and remits within a few weeks. It may occur with no apparent antecedent, but it may occur in the setting of head trauma, encephalitis, or CNS neoplasia. Presumably, focal CNS damage is responsible, but the EEG exhibits a generally slow background rhythm without focal spikes or sharp waves. Episodes may occur more than once, but they invariably cease before the patient is 30 years old.

## Klüver-Bucy Syndrome

With bilateral temporal lobe damage, male primates exhibit a syndrome of heightened distractibility, increased docility, visual agnosia, and inappropriate sexual activity. The hypersexual behavior consists of excessive, unconcealed masturbation and indiscriminate attempts at sexual intercourse with both male and female partners. Oral contact with the environment is excessive to the point of being dangerous to the patient. The patient will put sharp objects, feces, corrosive fluids, and other dangerous items in the mouth to investigate them.

The behavior patterns characteristic of Klüver-Bucy syndrome arise with damage to the mesiobasal temporal lobe, probably as a result of damage to the hippocampus, amygdala, and pyriform cortex. Damage occurring in these locations is usually irreversible. Tumors, infarction, contusions, encephalitis, and surgical resection are most likely to produce this damage.

## Priapism

Priapism is intractable erection. It may develop transiently in men with spinal cord disease or persistently in men with a variety of vascular disorders. It may develop also with hematologic disorders, such as sickle cell disease, thalassemia, and leukemia. Venous drains may relieve priapism before permanent penile damage occurs, but impotence is likely after priapism has remitted.

## BLADDER CONTROL

Bladder control is disturbed in many of the same disorders that affect sexual function. With damage to the lumbosacral spinal cord or cauda equina, the patient may develop a flaccid bladder. As the bladder fills beyond its capacity, the patient develops overflow incontinence. This may occur in diabetes mellitus, amyloidosis, and other causes of peripheral neuropathy. If the spinal cord is damaged above the lumbosacral level, bladder muscles usually become spastic. As the spastic bladder fills, premature contraction of the muscles produces urinary incontinence. This is usually the cause of incontinence in multiple sclerosis, subacute combined systems disease, and other diseases affecting the corticospinal tracts.

Enuresis, incontinence developing while the individual is asleep, may be an early sign of a seizure disorder. If it is associated with tongue-biting and convulsive limb movements, the diagnosis of seizures is fairly certain.

## SELECTED REFERENCES

Asbury AK: Understanding diabetic neuropathy. N Engl J Med *319*:577, 1988.

Beeley L: Drug-induced sexual dysfunction and infertility. Adverse Drug React Acute Poisoning Rev *3*:23, 1984.

Buffum J: Pharmacosexology: The effects of drugs on sexual function. J Psychoactive Drugs *14*:5, 1982.

Ellenberg M: Sexual function in diabetic patients. Ann Intern Med *92* (part 2):331, 1980.

Greydanus DE, Demarest DS, Sears JM: Sexual dysfunction in adolescents. Semin Adolescent Med *1*:177, 1985.

Kirkeby HJ, Poulsen EU, Petersen T, Dorup J: Erectile dysfunction in multiple sclerosis. Neurology *38*:1366, 1988.

Lechtenberg R: Multiple Sclerosis Fact Book. Philadelphia, F.A. Davis, 1988.

McGuire EJ: Myelodysplasia. Semin Neurol *8*:145, 1988.

Maruta T, Osborne D, Swanson DW, et al: Chronic pain patients and spouses: Marital and sexual adjustment. Mayo Clin Proc *56*:307, 1981.

Masters WH, Johnson VE: Human Sexual Response. Boston, Little, Brown and Company, 1980.

Mulligan T, Katz G: Erectile failure in the aged: Evaluation and treatment. J Am Geriatr Soc *36*:54, 1988.

Siroky MB: Neurophysiology of male sexual dysfunction in neurologic disorders. Semin Neurol *8*:137, 1988.

Smith PJ, Talbert RL: Sexual dysfunction with antihypertensives and antipsychotic agents. Clin Pharm *5*:373, 1986.

Strasberg PD, Brady SM: Sexual functioning of persons with neurologic disorders. Semin Neurol *8*:141, 1988.

*Chapter 9*

# Movement Disorders

Most movement disorders involve a decrease in activity, an increase in activity, or a profound aberration of activity. Many of the commonly occurring movement disorders develop with basal ganglia disease, which affects the caudate, putamen, globus pallidus, and substantia nigra.

## DECREASED MOVEMENT

Among the most common movement disorders are those which produce slower than normal movements. They are presumed to develop with impairment of neurons that use dopamine as their primary neurotransmitter. Acetylcholine may simplistically be considered the antagonist of dopamine, and much of the therapy for these types of movement disorders has attempted to increase dopamine levels or reduce acetylcholine levels at neural synapses in the brain.

### Parkinson Disease

Parkinson disease is an idiopathic cause of deterioration of the substantia nigra, with decreased mobility as one of its principal manifestations. In additon to slowing of movements, or bradykinesia, patients with Parkinson disease may exhibit tremors, rigidity, and dementia.

The most typical tremor appears when the patient is not moving and involves rhythmic flexion of the fingers (Table 9-1). This is called a pill-rolling tremor because the patient appears to be rolling a small object between his thumb and index finger. Tremors may involve the limbs more generally or even the trunk. Axial or head tremor that involves rhythmic flexion and extension of the spine is called titubation.

The rigidity associated with Parkinson disease may be lead-pipe or cogwheel, that is, continuous or stuttering. Inapparent cogwheel rigidity may be amplified by asking the patient to concentrate on a complex calculation while the examiner moves one of the patient's limbs passively. The cogwheel rigidity is felt as recurrent catches in the movement as part of the limb is moved about its joint.

Dementia often develops with Parkinson disease, but it may progress much less rapidly than the movement disorder and must be differentiated from depression that also develops with Parkinson disease.

Less consistently appearing signs of Parkinson disease include retropulsion, a tendency to fall backwards, and propulsion, a problem with arresting forward acceleration once it has begun. Neck

TABLE 9-1. *Tremors*

| Type | Activity | Character | Associated Diseases |
|---|---|---|---|
| Static | Rest | Rapid<br>Abates with voluntary movement | Parkinson disease<br>Drug-induced—phenothiazines<br>—butyrophenones<br>Wilson disease |
| Kinetic | Sustained posture<br>Voluntary movement | Slow<br>Low amplitude | Benign essential tremor<br>Drug-induced—caffeine<br>—lithium<br>—tricyclics<br>—amphetamines<br>—alcohol withdrawal<br>—opiate withdrawal<br>—isoproterenol<br>Mercury poisoning<br>Wilson disease<br>Hyperthyroidism<br>Cerebellar disease |
| Endpoint | Voluntary movement | Slow<br>Amplitude increases as target is approached | |

stiffness may be as substantial in individuals with Parkinson disease as it is in those with meningitis. Weight loss often develops with impaired appetite. The tremor that is evident when the patient is at rest or is sustaining a posture abates when a movement is initiated. This is called a sustention tremor, as opposed to a kinetic tremor, because it is typically not apparent during movements.

The affected individual's facial expression appears flat or masked, except when strong emotions induce reflex changes in expression. Spontaneous blinking is decreased, but reflex blinking on glabellar tapping is exaggerated and irrepressible.

Current management of Parkinson disease entails the use of a variety of anticholinergic and dopaminergic drugs (Table 9-2). A combination of L-dopa and carbidopa, a dopa decarboxylase inhibitor that crosses the blood-brain barrier very poorly, is the most commonly used antiparkinsonian therapy. Sinemet is one formulation of this combination that is currently available. The usual starting dose is 1 tablet of a 10/100 formulation (10 mg carbidopa with 100 mg L-dopa) 2 or 3 times a day. Dopamine cannot be given because it does not cross the blood-brain barrier. L-Dopa is converted in the central nervous system to dopamine. Carbidopa blocks the conversion of L-dopa to dopamine outside the central nervous system. High doses of L-dopa produce vomiting and hallucinations in many patients. Alternative formulations of carbidopa/L-dopa contain 25/100 and 25/250 doses. The size and frequency of doses must be determined on an individual basis, but most patients do not tolerate or benefit from more than 2 25/250 pills 4 times daily.

Alternative dopaminergic treatments include bromocriptine and lisuride. Bromocriptine (Parlodel) is available as 2.5-mg pills and may be taken as often as 4 times daily. Higher doses may be tolerated by the patient, but a levelling off of the therapeutic effect of the drug usually occurs at a lower dose. Lisuride is not generally available.

Anticholinergic treatments include trihexyphenidyl hydrochloride (Artane) and benztropine mesylate (Cogentin). The tricyclic antidepressants imipramine hydrochloride (Tofranil) and amitriptyline hydrochloride (Elavil) also have anticholinergic effects, but their

TABLE 9-2.   *Antiparkinsonian Drugs*

| Drug | Dosage | Frequency |
|------|--------|-----------|
| Carbidopa/L-dopa | 10 mg/100 mg | 3 or more times daily |
| | 25/100 | 3 or more times daily |
| | 25/250 | 3 or more times daily |
| Imipramine | 50 to 150 mg | once daily |
| Amitriptyline | 10 to 50 mg | once daily |
| Trihexyphenidyl | 2.5 mg | 1 to 3 times daily |
| Benztropine | 0.5 mg | 1 to 3 times daily |
| Amantadine | 100 mg | 1 to 2 times daily |
| Deprenyl | 5 mg | 2 times daily |
| α-Tocopherol | 2000 IU | once daily |

antiparkinsonian actions may have a broader basis than the anticholinergic effects alone. Amantadine hydrochloride (Symmetrel), an antiviral agent, has produced short-term benefits for many patients who have been given relatively low doses of the drug, but the basis for these antiparkinsonian effects is unknown. Drugs more recently introduced as antiparkinsonian agents, such as deprenyl (Eldepryl) and α-tocopherol, which are presumed to have antioxidant effects, appear to slow the progression of early Parkinson disease by inhibiting substantia nigra deterioration. In clinical trials, deprenyl and α-tocopherol have been used at doses of 5 mg twice a day and 2000 IU daily, respectively, but the ideal dosages of these drugs have yet to be firmly established.

Transplantation of adrenal or embryonal tissue into the brain has had remarkably variable effects. Most well documented cases have revealed slight or transient effects of the cell implants into the lateral ventricles or the basal ganglia. In many patients, the implanted cells fail to survive for more than a few weeks. The value of fetal tissue implants is still under study.

## Postencephalitic Parkinsonism

Signs of parkinsonism may develop after viral encephalitis. This was seen most commonly during the worldwide epidemic of encephalitis lethargica that lasted from 1918 to 1926. Postencephalitic parkinsonism still occurs, with the most directly implicated agent being the influenza virus. Before the rigidity and bradykinesia of parkinsonism develop, the affected individual may exhibit uncontrollable jerking or writhing movements of the limbs. As the involuntary movements abate, the parkinsonism becomes apparent. Very young people may be affected by this type of movement disorder. They may be treated with antiparkinsonian medications, but the outlook is generally poor for long-term improvement.

## Neuroleptic-Induced Parkinsonism

One of the most common types of parkinsonism is neuroleptically induced. Phenothiazines and butyrophenones may cause parkinsonian symptoms when used at the doses usually needed to manage psychotic disorders. These same drugs may also induce movement disorders characterized by excessive involuntary movements, but both complications of the drugs are usually transient. Parkinsonism will usually be evident, if it is going to appear at all, after the patient has taken the medications for 2 to 4 weeks. Haloperidol (Haldol) and the piperazine class of phenothiazines, of which trifluoperazine (Stelazine) is a member, are most likely to produce parkinsonism, whereas piperidine phenothiazines, such as thioridazine (Mellaril) and clozapine, are least likely. Anticholinergic medications, such as benztropine and trihexyphenidyl, are preferred over dopaminergic drugs, such as carbidopa/L-dopa and bromocriptine, to reduce the parkinsonian side effects of the drugs, because the dopaminergic drugs often exacerbate the psychiatric problems for which the neuroleptics were given.

## Wilson Disease (Hepatolenticular Degeneration)

Wilson disease is a recessively inherited disorder of copper metabolism characterized by damage to many organs, including the liver and the brain. The brain structures most obviously damaged are the putamen and globus pallidus of the basal ganglia, which together constitute the lenticular nuclei. Copper deposits in Descemet's membrane, on the posterior aspect of the cornea, produce a pigment ring that is usually apparent on slit-lamp examination of the eye. This Kayser-Fleischer ring is a reliable indicator of central nervous system involvement by Wilson disease. Renal tubular acidosis and cirrhosis may develop as other complications.

The neurologic signs of Wilson disease are variable and include parkinsonism, dementia, depression, and involuntary movements. The diversity of involuntary movements is substantial; consequently, any young adult with a movement disorder and hepatic dysfunction should be examined for Wilson disease. The diagnosis is based on increased levels of copper in the liver, increased excretion of copper in the urine, and abnormally low levels of ceruloplasmin in the blood. The level of ceruloplasmin is rarely normal with Wilson disease; but deficiency of this glycoprotein is not responsible for the disease, it is merely one facet of a multifaceted disorder. CT scans are almost always abnormal in patients with neurologic signs of Wilson disease. Ventricular enlargement is typical, with some associated cortical atrophy. The putamen and globus pallidus of the basal ganglia are usually obviously atrophied and hypodense. MR scanning of this area is even more diagnostic than CT because T2-weighted images reveal a characteristic enhancement of the globus pallidus and putamen.

The gene locus responsible for hepatolenticular degeneration is on chromosome 13. Current treatment focuses on reducing copper levels in the body. Intestinal copper absorption is normal in Wilson disease, but biliary elimination of copper is defective. Copper absorption may be reduced by avoiding copper-rich foods, such as chocolate, nuts, and lobster. The treatment of choice is a chelating agent, penicillamine, which reduces the load of copper the body must metabolize and thereby reduces the copper toxicity that accounts for some of the damage done by the disease. Fibrotic changes in the liver may be partially reversed by long-term treatment with penicillamine.

## Shy-Drager Syndrome

Shy-Drager syndrome is a degenerative disease that causes profound deterioration of the autonomic nervous system. It is associated with parkinsonian symptoms in many affected individuals, who are primarily men. Impotence is an early sign of dysautonomia in these men. The dysautonomia may progress to cause postural hypotension and other potentially lethal cardiovascular complications.

**Other Causes of Parkinsonism**

A variety of other conditions produces symptoms reminiscent of Parkinson disease. These include manganese poisoning, hyperparathyroidism, post-traumatic parkinsonism, idiopathic calcification of the basal ganglia, progressive supranuclear palsy (Steele-Richardson-Olszewski syndrome), and nonwilsonian hepatolenticular degeneration. Some of these conditions, such as manganese poisoning, may respond to levodopa treatment, but most do not.

## INCREASED MOVEMENT

Involuntary movements not associated with decreased motor activity occur even more commonly than does parkinsonism. This type of movement disorder may be limited to a habit spasm or tic producing excessive eye blinking, or it may involve many different muscle groups, thereby interfering with independent activity.

### Abnormal Facial Movements

The face is an especially common site for involuntary movements. Most patients with abnormal facial movements have habit spasms or drug-related movement disorders. Neuroleptic-associated dyskinesias are especially common in psychiatric patients treated with phenothiazines or butyrophenones for months or years. Occasionally, dyskinesias develop with limited exposure to neuroleptic drugs, but this is uncommon.

**Dyskinesias.** The individual with dyskinesias may have involuntary grimacing, opisthotonic posturing, tongue thrusting, and mouth opening. Diaphragmatic dyskinesias may produce grunting or gasping. These abnormal movements, like most abnormal movements, disappear with sleep.

The most common cause of dyskinesias is long-term use of neuroleptic agents. Idiosyncratic reactions to single doses of phenothiazines, butyrophenones, or even antihistamines may produce the same type of movement disorder. With these idiosyncratic reactions, the dyskinesias are less likely to be persistent than with long-term exposure to neuroleptics. The abnormal movements are sometimes called acute dystonic reactions, rather than dyskinesias, simply to differentiate them from the movement disorders associated with long-term administration of neuroleptics. Muscle tone is no more disturbed with acute dystonic reactions than it is with other dyskinesias.

The dyskinesias are presumed to arise with disturbed basal ganglia function, perhaps from hypersensitivity of dopamine receptors that were effectively denervated by long-term neuroleptic use. Imbalances in several neurotransmitters are probably involved in many patients with these dyskinesias.

Dyskinesias may be acute or tardive. The acute dyskinesias develop most often when neuroleptics are instituted or abruptly stopped. Movements typical of acute dyskinesias or dystonias include blepharospasm, oculogyric crisis, retrocollis, aversive eye movements, grimacing, slurred speech, and jaw clenching. If dyskinesias develop with drug withdrawal, they are often transient and abate completely within 5 weeks. This transient dyskinesia is presumed to be a manifestation of dopamine rebound after dopamine antagonists are withdrawn. Withdrawal-emergent dyskinesias most often occur with chlorpromazine (Thorazine) and thioridazine (Mellaril).

Dyskinesias may develop while the patient is still receiving long-term neuroleptics or they may persist for months or years after the neuroleptics are stopped. These are called tardive dyskinesias and are most often seen in elderly patients who have been receiving high-dose neuroleptics for several years. Severe tardive dyskinesia appears most commonly in those patients who exhibited pronounced parkinsonism when neuroleptic therapy was begun. Tardive dyskinesia most commonly involves the tongue or mouth and much less commonly affects the upper face than do acute dystonic reactions. Tongue writhing and thrusting, lip smacking, cheek puffing, and chewing movements are most typical of tardive dyskinesias. Limb and trunk movements may develop but are notably uncommon. Piperazine phenothiazines and butyrophenones are the drugs that most commonly produce tardive dyskinesias, and these dyskinesias rarely appear before the patient has been receiving the neuroleptic for less than 3 months. Tardive dyskinesias may remit with low-dose haloperidol treatment, an option that is unarguably less than ideal because the drug used to treat the disorder may be the original cause of the disorder. Bromocriptine and reserpine have been used to suppress tardive dyskinesias with some success, but both of these drugs may cause severe psychiatric reactions. Lithium and tricyclic antidepressants have also been effective in some individuals and pose less risk of psychiatric complications.

Tardive dyskinesia-like movements occasionally develop for no apparent reason. In one idiopathic syndrome called Meige's disease, blepharospasm is associated with oromandibular dyskinesia. This disorder usually appears in middle-aged adults or the elderly. Anticholinergic medications or haloperidol suppress the movements in some individuals.

## Focal Motor Seizures

Any paroxysmal involuntary movement should be evaluated as possible seizure activity. Partial seizures may appear as strictly motor phenomena, which may be little more than facial twitching or hand movements. If the results of an EEG support the diagnosis of focal motor seizure activity, the patient should be treated with an antiepileptic. Phenytoin (Dilantin) at 300 mg daily or carbamazepine (Tegretol) at 600 to 1200 mg daily should suppress the involuntary movement. Hemifacial spasms, in which involuntary contractions of one side of the face occur paroxysmally, are usually not from seizure activity and may be related to facial nerve damage. This type of focal movement disorder often remits spontaneously. The patient may have symptomatic relief with clonazepam (Klonopin) at 0.5 to 1.0 mg daily.

## Tooth Grinding (Bruxism)

Bruxism, the involuntary jaw movements that produce tooth grinding, commonly occurs during normal sleep. It is not truly a movement disorder, because at least 10% of the normal population has episodes of nocturnal tooth grinding. Malocclusion occasionally underlies the bruxism, but in most cases no pathologic processes are evident. If the movements are especially vigorous or forceful, teeth or dental work may be damaged. Individuals with this type of damage from grinding should be protected with a bite plate.

Bruxism that develops while an individual is awake may be a sign of progressive metabolic brain disease or evidence of phenothiazine or butyrophenone exposure. Tardive dyskinesia associated with neuroleptic use may start with bruxism.

## TREMORS

Tremors are rhythmic oscillations of the limbs or trunk. Rhythmic oscillations involving the head are called titubation. Tremors that appear during purposeful movements are kinetic tremors. Those that occur only when the patient is not engaged in a voluntary movement are called static or resting tremors. With Parkinson disease, an obvious resting tremor usually abates or disappears during voluntary movement of the affected limb. With cerebellar disease, the tremor becomes more apparent with voluntary limb movements, especially if substantial extension of the limb is involved. If the tremor becomes evident only with full extension of the limb, it is often referred to as an endpoint or intention tremor.

### Cerebellar Disease

Tremor is a common sign of cerebellar injury (Table 9-3). The tremor most often associated with cerebellar disease is the kinetic or intention tremor. It typically occurs in an extremity and often is ipsilateral to the site of cerebellar damage.

Lesions that develop routinely in the cerebellum range from infarction to demyelination. In multiple sclerosis, the cerebellum is

TABLE 9-3. *Signs and Symptoms of Focal Cerebellar Lesions*

| Signs | Symptoms |
| --- | --- |
| Gait ataxia | Headache |
| Limb and ocular dysmetria | Nausea and vomiting |
| Nystagmus | Gait difficulty |
| Dysdiadochokinesis | Vertigo or dizziness |
| Kinetic tremor | Diplopia |
| Dysarthria | Memory difficulty |
| Past-pointing | Blurred vision |
| Head tilt | Clumsiness |
| Abducens paresis | Tremor |
| Titubation | Tinnitus |
| Facial paresis | Dysphagia |
| Dysgraphia | |

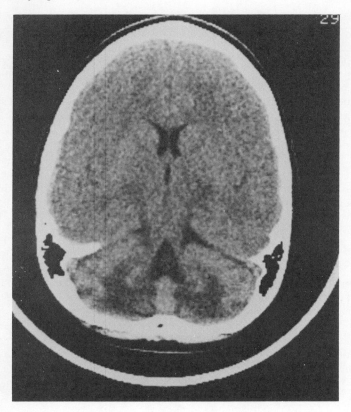

FIG. 9-1. This CT scan of a child with adrenoleukomyeloneuropathy, a rare hereditary disturbance of cerebellar myelination and adrenal function, associated with peripheral neuropathy and spinal cord disease, reveals decreased density in the cerebellar hemispheres in areas of dysmyelination. (With permission from Lechtenberg R: Seizure Recognition and Treatment. New York, Churchill Livingstone, 1990.)

an extroardinarily common site for demyelination, but similar lesions develop in several rare hereditary disorders (Fig. 9-1). Cerebellar atrophy occurs with many hereditary syndromes, most of which include tremor and gait ataxia as prominent symptoms. In many of the recessively inherited ataxias, the metabolic defect is known (Table 9-4).

**Essential Tremor**

A coarse tremor that is apparent at rest and persists during movements occurs as an inherited trait in some families. The tremor may worsen as the individual ages. Alcohol may decrease the severity of the tremor, a phenomenon that inclines some individuals to self-medicate with alcohol. The tremor is usually limited to the hands or arms. No lesions are apparent in the brains of affected individuals. Propranolol, atenolol, metoprolol, and other beta-blocking drugs may reduce the severity of the tremor if they are used chronically.

TABLE 9-4.  *Progressive Recessive Ataxias*

| Disease | Age at onset | Metabolic Defect |
|---------|--------------|------------------|
| Infantile Gaucher | 0–6 months | Glucosylceramidase deficiency |
| Sandhoff | 0–6 years | Hexosaminidase deficiency |
| Ataxia telangiectasia | 0–6 years | Unknown |
| Friedreich | 6–16 years | Unknown |
| Refsum | 6–16 years | Defect in alpha oxidation |
| Bassen-Kornzweig | 6–16 years | Abetalipoproteinemia |

## Hyperthyroidism

Fine resting tremors may develop with hyperthyroidism. Treatment of the thyroid disease usually reduces the tremor.

## TICS (HABIT SPASMS)

Tics are brief, repetitive, involuntary movements or sounds that interrupt otherwise normal activity. Characteristically, they may be suppressed voluntarily only with substantial attention and effort, and they recur with relaxation.

### Idiopathic Tics

The most common tics are eyeblinks, shoulder shrugs, head tosses, and facial grimaces. Vocal tics include grunts, sniffles, and throat clearing. More complex movements and vocalizations may occur, but they are considerably less common.

### Gilles de la Tourette Syndrome

Tourette syndrome involves multiple motor tics and vocal tics. The disorder appears before the individual is 21 years of age and persists for more than 1 year. The vocal tics usually include involuntary obscene, scatologic, or alarming words. The motor tics may involve fairly complex activities, such as combined arm and leg movements.

Men are more commonly affected than are women. The disorder is probably transmitted in an autosomal dominant pattern with variable penetrance.

If the symptoms of the disorder are disabling, the patient may profit from haloperidol at doses of 0.25 to 2.5 mg daily as a single dose. Alternative medications include trifluoperazine and fluphenazine. Pimozide at doses of 1.5 to 10 mg daily has been useful in patients who have excessive sedation with butyrophenone or phenothiazine treatment.

## CHOREA AND ATHETOSIS

Involuntary movements of the limbs and trunks include jerking and writhing. The more rapid movements are called choreiform and the slower are athetoid. Choreiform movements or chorea are some-

Jankovic J, Tolosa E (eds): Parkinson's Disease and Movement Disorders. Baltimore, Urban and Schwarzenberg, 1988.

Koller WC, Vetere-Overfield B: Acute and chronic effects of propranolol and primidone in essential tremor. Neurology *39*:1587, 1989.

Kurlan R: Tourette's syndrome: Current concepts. Neurology *39*:1625, 1989.

Lechtenberg R: The Psychiatrist's Guide to Diseases of the Nervous System. New York, John Wiley and Sons, 1982.

Marsden CD, Fahn S (eds): Movement Disorders. 2nd Ed. London, Butterworth, 1987.

Mas JL, Guegen B, Bouche P, et al: Chorea and polycythaemia. J Neurol *232*:169, 1985.

The Parkinson Study Group: Effect of deprenyl on the progression of disability in early Parkinson's disease. N Engl J Med *321*:1364, 1989.

Sax DS, Bird ED, Gusella JF, Myers RH: Phenotypic variation in two Huntington's disease families with linkage to chromosome 4. Neurology *39*:1332, 1989.

Shoulson I, Fahn S, Oakes D, et al: DATATOP: A multicenter controlled clinical trial in early Parkinson's disease. Arch Neurol *46*:1052, 1989.

Zweig RM, Koven SJ, Hedreen JC, et al: Linkage to the Huntington's disease locus in a family with unusual clinical and pathological features. Ann Neurol *26*:78, 1989.

## Chapter 10
# Sleep Disorders

Sleep may be excessive, insufficient, or interrupted by abnormal phenomena. A variety of activities, such as sleeptalking, tooth-grinding, and nocturnal emissions, may occur as normal variants during sleep. Normal sleep has several well-characterized phases, the elimination of which may produce cognitive and affective disturbances.

### SLEEP STAGES

Electroencephalographic and other types of physiologic studies have defined two types of sleep, rapid eye movement (REM) sleep and nonrapid eye movement (NREM) sleep. NREM sleep may be further divided into four electroencephalographically distinct stages. As the patient progresses through each stage of NREM sleep, the stimulus needed to wake the patient increases. In REM sleep, the arousal threshold is even higher than during NREM sleep, and yet the electroencephalogram has paradoxically alert features. It is during REM sleep that dreams occur. Less structured perceptions, such as night terrors, may occur during NREM sleep.

NREM sleep stages follow one another for about an hour before REM sleep is reached. The delay from NREM sleep to REM sleep may be considerably shortened if the patient has been sleep deprived or REM-sleep deprived. As the patient becomes drowsy, generalized slowing of the EEG appears. The alpha-wave patterns evident during relaxed wakefulness become more fragmented. This is stage 1 NREM sleep (Table 10-1).

Stage 2 is characterized by the appearance of 12 to 14 Hz sinusoidal waves, called sleep spindles, and high-voltage sharp waves about the vertex of the head. Combinations of sharp and slow-wave patterns appearing during NREM sleep are called K complexes.

Stage 3 occurs as sleep spindles become more evident and slowing of the EEG to delta rhythms takes over 20 to 50% of the recording. The delta activity increases to higher voltages and accounts for more than 50% of the EEG recording in stage 4 NREM sleep.

In REM sleep, the EEG abruptly records low amplitude fast activity as the predominant wave form. Muscle tone decreases and body movements, other than eye movements and breathing, largely disappear. Respiratory and cardiac rates vary considerably more during REM sleep than during NREM sleep. Men and boys with intact genital innervation have penile erections, and individuals of both sexes dream during REM sleep. The REM period usually lasts about 15 minutes and recurs several times nightly.

TABLE 10-1.  *Characteristics of Sleep Stages*

| Sleep Stages | EEG Changes | Eye Movements |
|---|---|---|
| Stage 1 | Interrupted alpha activity<br>Generalized slowing<br>No spindles | Slow |
| Stage 2 | Diffuse theta activity<br>Spindles and K complexes<br>Low-voltage background | Slow |
| Stage 3 | High-voltage slow waves<br>Occasional spindles<br>Delta activity during less than<br>half the recording | Slow |
| Stage 4 | High-voltage delta waves over<br>more than half the recording | Slow |
| REM | Low-voltage beta and theta waves | Rapid |

## DREAMS AND NIGHT TERRORS

The night terror, or pavor nocturnus, differs from the dream or nightmare in that it is an isolated image that frightens and often awakens the individual (Table 10-2). The patient may scream as he awakens and often has no recall of what the specific nature of the night terror was. Nightmares or incubi can usually be recalled if the patient awakens during them. The night terror occurs during NREM sleep; the incubus is usually if not always a feature of REM sleep. Children have night terrors much more commonly than do adults. Parkinsonian patients who are receiving levodopa may experience night terrors, but most report extremely vivid dreams, rather than typical night terrors.

Profoundly disturbing nightmares may be suppressed with tricyclic compounds, such as imipramine (Tofranil) at 100 mg nightly or amitriptyline (Elavil) at 25 mg nightly. Night terrors usually abate with low-dose diazepam (Valium) at bedtime.

## EFFECTS OF AGING AND STRESS

Sleep duration usually decreases with age, whereas the delay in sleep onset usually increases. The durations of stage 3 and stage 4 NREM sleep decreases with age. Sleep deprivation at any age increases the amount of stage 3 and stage 4 NREM sleep occurring on the first night of sleep recovery. REM sleep also usually increases

TABLE 10-2.  *Characteristics of Nightmares and Night Terrors*

| Nightmare | Night Terror |
|---|---|
| Frightening dream sequence | Frightening image |
| Agitated on awakening | Screams on awakening |
| Common in adults | Most common in children |
| Slight autonomic response | Profound autonomic response |
| Occurs during REM sleep | Occurs during stage 3 and 4 NREM sleep |
| Usually in late evening | Usually in early evening |
| Usually dream content recalled | Usually amnesic for specific features |
| Males and females equally susceptible | Males more susceptible |
| Unrelated to somnambulism | Often associated with somnambulism |

in individuals who are sleep deprived, but this compensatory change may not be evident until the second or third night after the deprivation.

## INSOMNIA

Insomnia includes decreased sleep duration, delayed sleep onset, and recurrent awakening during sleep. Stimulant-drug abuse and withdrawal from a variety of drugs may produce insomnia. This is true for alcohol, as well as for more obviously stimulant drugs, such as cocaine and amphetamines.

Sleep apnea interrupts normal sleep and produces excessive lethargy and napping during what should be periods of normal wakefulness. The patient awakens as his or her airway becomes obstructed. This problem usually arises in obese people.

Chronic depression may also produce sleeplessness, but problems with falling asleep, as well as with staying asleep, are usually evident. After barbiturate withdrawal, a patient may not recover a normal sleep pattern for several days. Patients with unexplained insomnia may improve with benzodiazepine drugs, such as chlordiazepoxide (Librium), administered at bedtime, but using any type of sleep medication increases the risk of developing drug dependence.

## HYPERSOMNIA

Endocrinologic and metabolic problems, such as hypothyroidism, hyperparathyroidism, diabetes mellitus, uremia, hypercalcemia, and hyperglycemia may produce excessive drowsiness and prolonged periods of sleep. Abuse of opiates, barbiturates, benzodiazepines, antihistamines, or other depressant drugs may produce excessive sleepiness that remains unexplained until toxicologic studies reveal the patient's surreptitious use of the drugs. Less readily corrected causes of hypersomnia include central nervous system disorders of sleep regulation. Subcortical tumors, encephalitis, or hydrocephalus may induce lethargy. Brainstem infarction secondary to mesencephalic artery occlusion may produce unremitting hypersomnia. Sepsis, dehydration, or anemia may produce little more than profound lethargy in the elderly before autonomic collapse occurs.

### Narcolepsy

Recurrent sleep attacks may be associated with cataplexy, hypnagogic hallucinations, and sleep paralysis in the idiopathic disorder called narcolepsy. The sleep attacks characteristically produce REM-onset sleep with each episode. Cataplexy, or loss of all postural tone, occurs while the patient is awake. Sleep paralysis is usually evident just after the patient awakens and makes it impossible for the patient to get out of bed. As the patient falls asleep, vivid hallucinations may develop. Occasionally, these are hypnopompic, that is, occurring as the patient awakens. The association of any of these three clinical phenomena with sleep attacks helps to confirm

the diagnosis of narcolepsy. Stimulant drugs, such as methylphen-
idate (Ritalin), may suppress sleep attacks, but cataplexy, sleep
paralysis, and hypnagogic hallucinations may respond more to tricyclic drugs, such as imipramine or clomipramine.

### Kleine-Levin Syndrome

Adolescent men who develop periodic hypersomnia in association
with excessive eating have the Kleine-Levin syndrome. Hypersexuality, bulimia, labile affect, and generalized hyperactivity commonly develop as part of the syndrome. Symptoms may remit as
the patient ages.

### Pickwickian Syndrome

Obese individuals may have sleep attacks with none of the other
clinical characteristics of narcolepsy. This is considered the Pick-
wickian syndrome if the patient has hyperphagia and idiopathic
hyperventilation. Arterial blood gases characteristically have an elevated $Pco_2$ and a depressed $Po_2$. Polycythemia and right ventricular
hypertrophy of the heart are also commonly present. The hypersomnia usually remits when the obesity is eliminated.

## ABERRANT BEHAVIOR DURING SLEEP

Some nocturnal activities are unusual, but not necessarily pathologic. Bruxism (tooth-grinding) during sleep occurs in about one
tenth of the population, but tongue biting associated with bruxism
may be evidence of seizure activity. Nocturnal emissions often occur
in young men in or about puberty. Their occurrence or absence is
not abnormal. Nocturnal bedwetting (enuresis) is worrisome in adults
with no structural bladder or sphincter problems, but is neither
worrisome nor significant in children who have no other neurologic
or psychiatric symptoms.

### Somnambulism

Sleepwalking as well as sleeptalking (somniloquy) occur during
stage 2 or 4 NREM sleep. They may be confused with complex
partial seizures unless experience with other affected family mem-
bers has revealed the benign nature of the nocturnal activity. Nocturnal enuresis occurs in the same families exhibiting a high incidence of somnambulism, but the basis for either sleep anomaly is
unknown. The somnambulist may appear awake and fearful during
the excursion, but he or she will be amnesic for the episode. Children
exhibit this behavior much more commonly than do adults. A 24-
hour EEG recording will help distinguish the sleep anomaly from
the seizure disorder. Even if seizure activity is not evident, antiepileptic medications, such as phenytoin and carbamazepine, may
suppress the behavior.

## Enuresis

Nocturnal bedwetting (enuresis) may be the first sign of seizure activity or spinal cord disease, but idiopathic enuresis also occurs during stage 4 NREM sleep. If seizure or spinal cord problems are not responsible, imipramine or amitriptyline treatment may suppress the bladder emptying.

## Restless Legs

Disagreeable sensations in the legs when the patient is supine may oblige the patient to stand and walk before successfully getting to sleep. Ischemia in the legs may contribute to this discomfort in some patients. In many individuals, no pathologic changes in the legs are evident. Exercise may be useful in suppressing the discomfort. If involuntary limb jerks are a prominent component of the restlessness, clonazepam 0.5 mg 1 to 3 times daily may eliminate the problem.

## SELECTED REFERENCES

Asbury AK, McKhann GM, McDonald WI (eds): Diseases of the Nervous System. Clinical Neurobiology. Philadelphia, W.B. Saunders, 1986.

Karacan I, Moore CA, Williams RL: The narcoleptic syndrome. Psychiatr Ann 9:69, 1979.

Kramer M: Dream disturbances. Psychiatr Ann 9:50, 1979.

Lechtenberg R: The Psychiatrist's Guide to Diseases of the Nervous System. New York, John Wiley, 1982.

Schachter M, Parkes JD: Fluvoxamine and clomipramine in the treatment of cataplexy. J Neurol Neurosurg Psychiatr 43: 71, 1980.

Ware JC: The symptom of insomnia: Causes and cures. Psychiatr Ann 9:27, 1979.

# Chapter 11
# Weakness

Weakness may be congenital, progressive, or acute. Each type of weakness may be from a variety of causes, including hereditary, infectious, toxic, and metabolic. The course and character of the weakness usually suggest its origin.

## MUSCULAR DYSTROPHY

Hereditary weakness of skeletal muscles develops with a variety of genetic defects. The gene affected may be in the nuclear or mitochondrial chromatin. Treatments are currently unavailable for these muscular dystrophies, but their genetic bases are being rapidly elucidated. Gene repair or protein replacements may soon provide feasible solutions to these disorders.

### Duchenne Dystrophy

Duchenne dystrophy is caused by a defect in the gene responsible for producing dystrophin, a protein essential for the normal functioning of skeletal muscles. This is inherited in a sex-linked recessive manner, consequently producing symptoms in young boys rather than in girls. The children affected usually have mild retardation as well as progressive weakness. They are usually wheelchair-bound by the time they are 11 years old. Muscle samples reveal less than 3% of the normal dystrophin content.

### Becker's Variant

Before the elucidation of the genetic basis for Duchenne dystrophy, adults with progressive weakness evolving in a similar pattern but without the early lethality of Duchenne dystrophy were recognized. The gene involved in these adults is also that responsible for the manufacture of dystrophin, but the muscle content of dystrophin is greater than 3% of the normal level. At what age weakness first appears and to what degree the patient has progressive weakness are determined by how much normal dystrophin his abnormal chromatin produces. Severe Becker dystrophy may be symptomatic in adolescence, but the disease is more typically the cause of progressive weakness later in life.

### Myotonic Dystrophy

Myotonia is a disturbance of muscle relaxation. Individuals with myotonia have persistent contractions of muscles. Typically, the affected individual reports that he cannot let go of the steering wheel after driving for a few minutes or he cannot put down a book that he was holding. Tapping a muscle may be a sufficient stimulus to elicit an involuntary and protracted contraction. Patients with this muscle disorder are invariably weak.

The most common hereditary form of myotonia is myotonic dystrophy, an autosomal recessive disorder. Affected individuals develop weakness, muscle wasting, cataracts, and heart blocks as adults. Men with this disorder have testicular atrophy and early baldness. Affected women may have menopause early in adult life. The EMG reveals a characteristic pattern of repetitive discharges with minor stimulation.

The cause of myotonic dystrophy is unknown, but the pattern of deficits suggests that this is a myopathy with a metabolic basis. No treatment is available for the weakness associated with this disorder, but patients may profit from pacemaker placement and symptomatic management of the myotonia with quinidine or procainamide.

## TRANSIENT WEAKNESS

Focal limb, facial, or ocular motor weakness may develop with transient ischemic attacks (Table 11-1). The pattern of weakness and associated neurologic deficits defines the part of the nervous system impaired. A transient right hemiparesis associated with a right hemisensory deficit implicates the motor and sensory cortex of the left cerebral hemisphere. A pure right hemiparesis without associated sensory problems may arise with ischemia to the left internal capsule. More focal weakness may transiently appear with restricted injuries to muscular innervation. For example, a traction injury of the brachial plexus may produce weakness in the major groups of the arm. Poisons, such as curare or botulinum, may reversibly block the neuromuscular junction and produce transient weakness affecting both the limbs and the diaphragm.

## FACIAL WEAKNESS

Weakness primarily of the lower face is usually associated with a lesion in the cerebral cortex or internal capsule. The eye on the weak side may have a slightly enlarged interpalpebral fissure because of relatively poor tone in the orbicularis oculi contralateral to the cerebral injury. Both sides of the cerebral cortex exert some control over the facial muscles of the ipsilateral and contralateral forehead. If weakness is evident over the upper and lower face on

TABLE 11-1. *Causes of Transient Weakness*

Transient ischemic attacks
Focal motor seizures
Hemiplegic migraine
Hysterical conversion reaction
Local trauma
Transient electrolyte abnormalities
Neuromuscular junction poisons

one side, the patient probably has a lesion in the brainstem damaging the facial nerve nucleus or an injury directly to cranial nerve VII. Bilateral facial weakness is characteristic of myasthenia gravis, progressive myopathies, or other causes of generalized weakness.

## Hemifacial Weakness

Facial weakness may develop with a hemiparesis or independently. In facial weakness from a cerebrocortical event, the forehead is spared because of bilateral control in each cerebral hemisphere. With damage to the facial nucleus or facial nerve, both lower and upper halves of the face are affected.

Common causes of facial weakness include tumors, such as schwannomas, on the facial nerve and basilar meningitides, such as tuberculosis, producing inflammation around the cranial nerve. With Lyme borreliosis, the facial nerve is especially likely to be impaired if neuroborreliosis develops. Lesions in the parotid gland may impinge on the facial nerve and produce weakness.

## Bell's Palsy

Idiopathic damage to the facial nerve is usually called Bell's palsy. The patient often has considerable discomfort just behind the ear where the facial nerve exits the stylomastoid foramen. Hemifacial paralysis may evolve over the course of hours or days with Bell's palsy. Patients with diabetes mellitus and other causes of progressive neuropathy are often left with some permanent weakness as this inflammatory disorder of the facial nerve abates. High-dose steroids are usually given to individuals with Bell's palsy, but only for 10 days to 2 weeks, with the dose of steroid tapered rapidly over the course of treatment. Symptoms usually associated with Bell's palsy include changes in taste and hearing. Taste may be impaired perceptibly on one side of the tongue from damage to the chorda tympani. Because the stapedius muscle is controlled by fibers from the facial nerve, damage to the facial nerve may produce hypersensitivity to noises from laxity of the stapedius muscle. The facial nerve damage presumably is caused by a viral infection.

## Lyme Disease

Lyme disease has recently become a relatively common cause of acute hemifacial weakness. It is caused by a spirochete Borrelia burgdorferi, which is carried by the deer tick Ixodes dammini. Tick bites spread the infection to people. A rash, erythema chronica migrans, may be an early indication of infection with the organism, but chronic problems with joint, cardiac, and neurologic disease may appear even if the rash does not.

Individuals with facial weakness caused by neuroborreliosis often have pleocytosis in the CSF. MR scans may reveal plaques of demyelination in individuals with chronic disease. The special susceptibility of the facial nerve to injury is unexplained. Patients with the neuroborreliosis of Lyme disease should be treated with meningitic doses of penicillin or ceftriaxone.

## GENERALIZED WEAKNESS

Progressive generalized weakness develops with metabolic disorders, primary muscle disease, primary nerve disease, or neuromuscular junction disorders. Drugs can induce paralysis, but the drugs responsible, which include curare and decamethonium, are difficult to administer surreptitiously outside a medical facility. Nerve or muscle disease may develop secondary to an infectious agent: diphtheria often gives rise to a polyneuropathy; many viral infections cause polymyositis.

### Myasthenia Gravis and Myasthenic Syndromes

Myasthenia denotes muscle weakness and easy fatigability associated with abnormalities at the neuromuscular junction. Myasthenia gravis develops with autoimmune damage to the acetylcholine receptor of noncardiac striated muscle. Patients complain of generalized weakness or blurred vision. With progression of the disorder, the patient may develop impaired breathing from diaphragmatic weakness or dysphagia from weakness in the upper third of the esophagus. Heart, bladder, and bowel musculature are all unaffected.

The muscles most consistently exhibiting weakness are the extrinsic muscles of the eye. Results of electrical studies of other muscles usually show a typical pattern of response to repetitive stimulation. The muscle action potentials recorded usually decrease in amplitude when the nerve to the muscle studied is repetitively stimulated at a rate of 25 to 50 shocks per second. The decrease in amplitude of the action potential after repetitive stimulation for 1 or 2 seconds should be more than 15% if the cause of the patient's weakness is myasthenia gravis.

Myasthenia gravis responds to several types of treatment (Table 11-2). The simplest is anticholinesterase medication. By blocking the action of cholinesterase at the neuromuscular junction, these drugs prolong the effect of acetylcholine that does find receptors

TABLE 11-2.  *Treatment of Myasthenia Gravis*

| Modality | Latency of Effect |
| --- | --- |
| Anticholinesterase | |
|    Edrophonium chloride | Seconds to minutes |
|    Pyridostigmine bromide | Minutes to hours |
| Corticosteroids | |
|    Prednisone | Days to weeks |
|    Thymectomy | Months to years |
| Cytotoxic immunosuppressants | |
|    Azathioprine | 4 to 6 months |
|    Cyclophosphamide | 2 to 6 weeks |
| Plasmapheresis | Minutes |

with which to bind. Edrophonium (Tensilon) is a rapidly acting anticholinesterase that is often useful in helping to establish the diagnosis of myasthenia gravis. After a dose of 0.4 to 1.0 mg, the affected patient may exhibit improved strength for a few minutes. The drug exerts a visible effect within seconds of intravenous administration, but it causes profound autonomic effects, such as hypotension, salivation, and gastrointestinal distress, which make it impractical for all but diagnostic applications. Slower onset, longer acting anticholinesterases, such as pyridostigmine, are useful therapeutically, but they too are limited by their cholinergic side effects, which include diarrhea and diaphoresis.

Thymectomy, the partial or complete resection of thymic tissue from the mediastinum, has a slowly appearing effect on the course of myasthenia gravis. About 50 to 70% of patients subjected to thymectomy improve over the course of 1 to 5 years. This treatment was first adopted because many patients with thymomas had myasthenia gravis and many patients with myasthenia gravis had thymic hyperplasia. Patients with neither thymoma nor hyperplasia who have myasthenia gravis routinely experience a more benign course with their illness if the thymus is removed early in the disease.

Corticosteroids, such as prednisone, are very effective in reducing the severity of myasthenic symptoms, but the long-term side effects of these drugs, which include diabetes mellitus, hypertension, and cataracts, limit their usefulness. Patients given prednisone experience improvement or remission of myasthenic symptoms in 80% of cases. Transient worsening of symptoms complicates the first few weeks of treatment.

Plasmapheresis, in which plasma laden with antiacetylcholine-receptor antibodies is filtered, may provide transient improvement of the myasthenia, but has no long-term benefits. This is also true of plasma exchange. These plasma manipulations may, however, be useful in patients with an acute myasthenic crisis that is refractory to other antimyasthenic measures. Cytotoxic immunosuppressants have been used with some success. Azathioprine is one antimetabolite that has been widely used. It exhibits an effect after many months and is primarily useful as an adjunctive therapy that allows reduction of the steroid dose needed to maintain the patient in remission. Cyclophosphamide is much more effective than azathioprine in inducing improvement or remission, but its side effects, which include hemorrhagic cystitis, limit its application. Cyclosporine has been used in limited trials and may prove useful in the future.

Other myasthenic syndromes may develop with damage to the neuromuscular junction presynaptically or with production of acetylcholine packets for delivery across the neuromuscular junction. The most common myasthenic syndrome is the Eaton-Lambert syndrome. This usually develops in patients with lung cancer and is associated with proliferative changes in the cell membranes of the neuromuscular junctions and with a characteristic electromyographic pattern in which muscle action potentials increase three- to fourfold in amplitude with repetitive stimulation (25 to 50 stimuli per second). The defect in presynaptic function is presumed to be from antibody interference with calcium channel operation.

TABLE 11-3.  *Causes of Myopathies*

| Class of Disease | Specific Diseases |
| --- | --- |
| Infectious | Viral polymyositis |
| Parasitic | Cysticercosis |
| Collagen | Dermatomyositis |
| vascular | Scleroderma |
| Idiopathic | Sarcoidosis |
| | Polymyalgia rheumatica |
| | Giant cell arteritis |
| Metabolic | Hypokalemia |
| Endocrinologic | Hyperthyroidism |
| | Hypothyroidism |
| Genetic defects | McArdle's phosphorylase deficiency |
| | Phosphofructokinase deficiency |
| | Mitochondrial myopathies |

A myasthenic picture also develops with tick paralysis. The tick responsible releases a paralyzing toxin after burrowing into the victim's skin. The treatment of tick paralysis is complete removal of the tick.

### Myopathies

Myopathies are intrinsic diseases of muscle arising from metabolic, hormonal, infectious, or other disorders (Table 11-3). Myopathy may be an imflammatory disease with numerous muscles affected, in which case it is called polymyositis. On a worldwide basis, polymyositis develops most commonly with infestation by the tapeworm Taenia solium, the cause of cysticercosis. Polymyositis in association with a violaceous periorbital rash (heliotrope rash) and erythema over the knuckles of the hands suggests dermatomyositis. Inflammatory muscle disease developing with noncaseating granulomas in multiple organs suggests sarcoidosis.

Results of the electromyogram (EMG) typically reveal abnormally small, irregularly formed action potentials and poor interference patterns. Affected muscles may be excessively irritable. A spontaneous action potential can be evoked by sticking a recording electrode into the muscle.

Some of the myopathies improve with corticosteroid treatment, but most are still untreatable.

### Neuropathies

Nerve damage may produce weakness independent of sensory deficits. Toxins such as lead may produce this type of neuropathy, but the most common cause of nonsensory neuropathy in the United States is diabetes mellitus. Diabetes mellitus may produce several different types of neuropathy in affected individuals. The four most commonly occurring types are symmetric sensory neuropathy, mononeuritis multiplex, diabetic amyotrophy, and dysautonomia. The symmetric sensory neuropathy produces a typical glove-and-stocking pattern of impaired pain, touch, and temperature perception. In mononeuritis multiplex, damage to individual nerves produces motor and sensory deficits in the distribution of the affected nerves. Diabetic amyotrophy may be associated with some pain, but it is typically a problem of limb girdle strength. Dysautonomia produces impotence, postural hypotension, and problems with gastrointestinal mobility.

The diseases most commonly causing neuropathies, such as diabetes mellitus, amyloidosis, leprosy, vitamin deficiency, systemic lupus erythematosus, and endocrine disturbances, usually produce a mixed sensory and motor neuropathy. Trauma to primarily motor nerves, such as the deep peroneal nerve, may produce little or no evidence of hypesthesias in association with the weakness.

## Guillain-Barré Syndrome

Landry-Guillain-Barré-Strohl syndrome is a rapidly progressive cause of skeletal muscle paralysis. Usually, patients develop weakness initially in the legs and subsequently in the arms and face. The weakness routinely evolves over 2 weeks or less and, at its worst, may completely suppress breathing. Ventilatory support becomes essential for survival. Affected individuals do not develop any ophthalmoplegia, except in rare variants of the syndrome. Sensory complaints are minimal or completely absent. Many patients complain of discomfort about their feet or lower legs, which may even precede the weakness. Bladder and bowel control are usually maintained despite the weakness that develops.

This was previously known as cytoalbuminemic dissociation because of the extremely high levels of protein developing in cerebrospinal fluid during the illness. Protein content in excess of 200 mg/dl is routine; occasionally, protein content exceeds 1 g/dl. This elevated protein is in sharp contrast to little or no increase in the cellular content of CSF.

The weakness often develops within a few weeks of a viral syndrome, but at the time the weakness appears, the patient is invariably afebrile. The absence of fever and presence of cytoalbuminemic dissociation helps distinguish this progressive paralysis from poliomyelitis.

Treatment for Guillain-Barré syndrome has been difficult to assess because of the variability of outcomes in patients with the disorder. Many individuals fully recover strength over the course of weeks or months. Others are left with residual paraparesis or paraplegia. Plasmapheresis has produced some improvement in the course if not the outcome of the disease.

## Poliomyelitis

Poliomyelitis is a motor neuron disease caused by a virus. The virus is spread by passage through the gastrointestinal tract. Individuals contracting the disease characteristically have a febrile illness with progressive weakness and cerebrospinal fluid signs of meningoencephalitis. Respiratory failure often develops as the disease progresses. Permanent weakness in isolated muscle groups, paraparesis, or paraplegia may occur if the patient survives the acute illness.

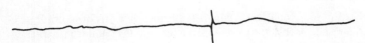

FIG. 11-1. With anterior horn-cell damage, the EMG records abnormally small, biphasic potentials, called fibrillations, from the muscle fibers innervated by the injured neuron. (From Lechtenberg R: The Psychiatrist's Guide to Diseases of the Nervous System. New York, John Wiley and Sons, 1982.)

### Amyotrophic Lateral Sclerosis (ALS)

Amyotrophic lateral sclerosis (ALS) is a motor neuron disease of unknown cause. Death occurs within months or years of the first symptoms, the rapidity of deterioration being related to how severely involved brainstem nuclei are early in the disease. Early signs of ALS include fasciculations, involuntary twitching of individual motor units. Results of the EMG reveal abnormally small muscle potentials, called fibrillations, developing spontaneously in the resting muscles (Fig. 11-1). MR studies of the spinal cord should reveal no focal injuries, but generalized atrophy may be apparent. No treatment has substantially affected the course of this disease.

### Werdnig-Hoffman and Related Motor Neuron Diseases

Congenital or early-onset motor neuron disease may produce profound weakness, hypotonia, and muscle atrophy in infants and children. The earliest onset and most lethal form of this damage to the motor system is Werdnig-Hoffman disease. Infants with this disease usually die. A similar pattern of motor neuron disease may become evident later in childhood. This is often called Kugelberg-Welander disease and does not carry the extreme lethality characteristic of Werdnig-Hoffman disease.

### Multiple Sclerosis

Weakness in a limb, or paraparesis, may be one of the earliest signs of multiple sclerosis. Because the weakness associated with multiple sclerosis is from demyelination of the corticospinal tracts, spasticity, hyper-reflexia, and positive Babinski signs routinely accompany any paraparesis or limb weakness. Bladder dysfunction is also commonly associated with the paraparesis of multiple sclerosis. Other problems often caused by multiple sclerosis include visual loss, gait ataxia, clumsiness, dysarthria, and easy fatigability.

Multiple sclerosis is usually described by the pattern and persistence of the neurologic problems that develop. If the patient has distinct episodes of rapid deterioration followed by gradual recovery of disrupted neurologic function, the disease is called remitting-relapsing. If the deterioration is inexorable and unremitting, the disease is called chronic progressive. Other categories of disease occur less commonly, but distinctions between various types of multiple sclerosis have been called into question by MR imaging of the

CNS in individuals with clinically distinct patterns of multiple sclerosis. The MR patterns of MS are remarkably similar in remitting-relapsing, chronic progressive, and other clinical subtypes of MS.

The diagnosis of multiple sclerosis usually requires observation over months or years. The association of problems in several different parts of the central nervous system appearing at different times, a phenomenon often described as lesions disseminated in space and time, is especially characteristic of multiple sclerosis. MR scanning may reveal plaques of demyelination scattered throughout the central nervous system, but the MR scanner cannot distinguish between demyelination from multiple sclerosis and that caused by viral infections, ischemia, or other diffuse CNS problems.

The lesion underlying all of these signs and symptoms is the plaque of demyelination. The myelin sheath created by the oligodendroglial cells in the CNS is stripped off the nerve fibers it insulates (Fig. 11-2). The cause of this demyelination is still unknown, but much evidence suggests an infectious basis for the disease. Inflammatory infiltrates are associated with the plaques of demyelination.

No treatment is truly effective, but prednisone or ACTH given at the time of flareups may shorten the acute phase of the illness. Because many immune system abnormalities are associated with multiple sclerosis, many therapeutic efforts have been directed at suppressing immune responses. Some studies suggest improved long-term outcomes with cyclophosphamide treatment, but the complications of this immunosuppressant therapy are substantial and include hemorrhagic cystitis and neutropenia. Trials with plasmapheresis have also improved clinical outcomes in some patients, but the advantages of and indications for this expensive modality are controversial.

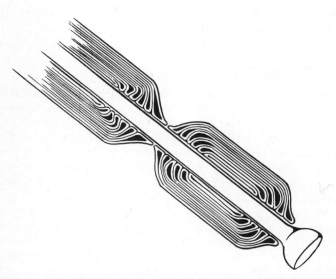

FIG. 11-2. This schematic depicts the normal structure of the myelin sheath around an axon. Two segments of sheath abut at the node of Ranvier. (With permission from Lechtenberg R: Multiple Sclerosis Fact Book. Philadelphia, F.A. Davis, 1988.)

## Brown-Sequard Syndrome

Hemisection of the spinal cord produces a characteristic pattern of neurologic deficits, which includes ipsilateral weakness and spasticity, ipsilateral loss of vibration and position sense, and contralateral loss of pain and temperature sensation. All of these problems are below the level of the spinal cord injury. Pain and temperature disturbances are three or four dermatomal levels below the cord level that is damaged. Fibers that conduct sensations of pain and temperature ascend a few cord segments before crossing over to form the spinothalamic tracts. Muscle atrophy may be evident at the level of injury if many anterior horn cells are damaged along with the long-tract damage.

Trauma and tumors are the most common causes of the Brown-Sequard syndrome. Recovery after transection of half the cord is usually negligible. If the syndrome resulted from a neurofibroma, meningioma, or other resectable spinal cord tumor, recovery of spinal cord function may be nearly complete.

## SELECTED REFERENCES

Adams CWM, Poston RN, Buk SJ: Pathology, histochemistry and immunochemistry of lesions in acute multiple sclerosis. J Neurol Sci 92:291, 1989.

Albers JW: AAEE case report #4: Guillain-Barré syndrome. Muscle Nerv 12:705, 1989.

Dupuis MJM: The spectrum of neurological manifestations of Borrelia burgdorferi infections. Rev Neurol 144:765, 1988.

Hoffman EP, Kunkel LM, Angelini C, et al: Improved diagnosis of Becker muscular dystrophy by dystrophin testing. Neurology 39:1011, 1989.

Gilman S, Winans SS: Manter and Gatz's Essentials of Clinical Neuroanatomy and Neurophysiology. 6th Ed. Philadelphia, F. A. Davis, 1982.

Jablecki CK, Berry C, Leach J: Survival prediction in amyotrophic lateral sclerosis. Muscle Nerv 12:833, 1989.

Koopmans RA, Li DKB, Oger JJF, et al: Chronic progressive multiple sclerosis: Serial magnetic resonance brain imaging over six months. Ann Neurol 26:248, 1989.

Kurtzke JF: Patterns of neurologic involvement in multiple sclerosis. Neurology 38:1235, 1989.

Mastalgia FL (ed): Inflammatory Diseases of Muscle. London, Blackwell, 1988.

Pachner AR, Duray P, Steere AC: Central nervous system manifestations of Lyme disease. Arch Neurol 46:790, 1989.

Rowland LP (ed): Merritt's Textbook of Neurology. 8th ed. Philadelphia, Lea & Febiger, 1989.

Sher E, Gotti C, Canal N, et al: Specificity of calcium channel autoantibodies in Lambert-Eaton myasthenic syndrome. Lancet 2:640, 1989.

Weiner HL, Dau PC, Khatri BO, et al: Double-blind study of true vs. sham plasma exchange in patients treated with immunosuppression for acute attacks of multiple sclerosis. Neurology 39:1143, 1989.

# Chapter 12
# Sensory Abnormalities

Sensory disturbances include pain secondary to progressive disease, pain with static lesions, and altered sensation from a variety of structural, inflammatory, and metabolic causes. The altered sensation may be an excessive sensitivity to tactile stimuli (hyperpathia), disturbed perceptions independent of tactile stimuli (paresthesia), impaired perception of stimuli (hypesthesia), and complete loss of sensory perception (anesthesia). Paresthesias are usually experienced as pins-and-needles sensations. If they are strictly painful, they are called dysesthesias.

## PAIN

Pain may be an indication of disease in innervated structures or an indication of damage to the nerve itself. Low back pain may be from a spinal root compressed by a herniated intervertebral disc or from a retroperitoneal mass. Cutting a nerve may produce chronic pain, such as that experienced with phantom limb pain, or eliminate all sensory perception, such as that achievable with an effective nerve block. Lesions in specific parts of the nervous system usually produce specific patterns of pain. With demyelinating spinal cord disease, such as that occurring with multiple sclerosis, the patient often has electrical sensations radiating down the spine with flexion of the neck (Lhermitte's sign). Patients with multiple sclerosis may also have spasms of muscle contractions that are extremely painful.

### Peripheral Neuropathy

Peripheral nerves are most commonly damaged with endocrinologic disturbances, such as diabetes mellitus, vitamin deficiency states, such as thiamine deficiency, and toxic injuries, such as insecticide poisoning. Thiamine deficiency usually produces painful neuropathy with hyperpathia and burning dysesthesias. Diabetes mellitus may cause paresthesias associated with hypesthesia. The pain associated with some peripheral neuropathies may be relieved with the antiepileptic drug carbamazepine or the tricyclic imipramine. In all peripheral neuropathies, the treatment of choice is correcting the underlying disorder if that is feasible.

**Causalgia.** Nerve injury without complete nerve destruction often occurs with bullet wounds and other high-velocity projectile injuries to a limb. A common consequence of this type of injury is intractable pain and hyperpathia. This type of neuropathy is called causalgia, and some evidence suggests that it is as much a disturbance of sympathetic nerve fibers as it is of pain fibers. Sympathetic nerve blocks have been useful in individuals with causalgia.

**Meralgia Paresthetica.**   The lateral femoral cutaneous nerve is an especially common site of peripheral nerve injury. It occurs in many obese, pregnant, or diabetic individuals and presents as paresthesias or dysesthesias over the anterior or lateral aspect of the upper thigh. This is called meralgia paresthetica and is usually self-limited. Weight loss may eliminate the problem in obese individuals.

**Carpal Tunnel Syndrome.**   With compression of the median nerve in the carpal tunnel, pain and paresthesias develop in the palm of the hand, especially about the thenar eminence. Compression often occurs with chronic trauma to the volar aspect of the wrist. Typists traditionally exhibit a high incidence of carpal tunnel syndrome. With hormonal disturbances, such as those associated with pregnancy, pituitary disorders, and thyroid disease, the median nerve is also susceptible to the carpal tunnel syndrome. With transient disturbances, such as pregnancy, the syndrome often remits spontaneously. Local injections of corticosteroids and splinting of the wrist also produce remission in many affected individuals. Those not helped by these maneuvers may require surgery to release the ligaments causing the compression of the median nerve.

**Shoulder-Hand Syndrome.**   Vasomotor tone is lost and pain develops in limbs immobilized for protracted intervals. A self-propagating pain syndrome commonly develops in the arm in patients with spinal root disease or even arm discomfort associated with myocardial infarctions. The problem appears to be in the sympathetic nerve fibers, and so the syndrome is often called reflex sympathetic dystrophy. Physical therapy and sympathetic ganglion blocks are helpful in reversing the syndrome.

## Low Back Pain

Low back pain arises from damage to bone, ligaments, nerves, or adjacent structures. If a spinal root compressed by a herniated intervertebral disc is the cause of the pain, the pain typically radiates down the leg along the distribution served by the injured root. An L5 radiculopathy may produce shooting pains down the inside of the leg to the great toe; an S1 root compression may produce pain down the back of the leg and into the lateral aspect of the foot. Even if typically radicular features appear, other causes of low back pain must be considered and investigated. In elderly men, this means that prostate or gastrointestinal cancer metastases to the bone must be considered. In women, ovarian or uterine tumors are likely to be responsible. Degenerative joint disease may cause pain for male or female patients, but the specific reason for the pain is usually suggested by x-ray findings. Low back pain should be investigated with routine x-rays of the lumbosacral spine, as well as careful physical examination to look for superficial problems. Women must have pelvic examinations as part of the evaluation. Men should have serum levels of prostatic-specific antigen and acid phosphatase checked. High levels suggest prostatic carcinoma. If a pelvic mass is likely, CT or MR imaging of the pelvis should be revealing. If a spinal root compression is more likely, CT or MR views of the spine may be helpful. A myelogram may be necessary to determine the character of the lesion.

Uncomplicated radiculopathies associated with disc herniation may respond to bedrest for 1 or 2 weeks. Pelvic traction is often applied to limit the patient's movement in bed and to assure that the patient remains flat. If the patient has developed substantial sensory or motor deficits or if a disc fragment is impinging on the root, surgery may be unavoidable. A laminectomy with disc resection is the surgery of choice.

### Thalamic Syndrome

With a pure sensory stroke, the patient has loss of sensation on the side of the body opposite the lesion. Occasionally, dysesthesias and hyperpathia develop over the area of sensory loss. This is called the thalamic syndrome because it usually develops after lacunar infarction of part of the thalamus. Tricyclic drugs, such as imipramine and amitriptyline, often suppress the pain experienced with this syndrome.

### Phantom Limb Pain

Searing or dull pain usually develops in a limb that has been amputated. The pain seems to arise in the member that has been removed and may persist for weeks, months, or years after the amputation. This phantom limb pain is usually refractory to a variety of treatments, including revision of the amputation site, sympathectomy, and analgesic medications. Biofeedback has been more helpful than other therapeutic approaches.

### PARESTHESIAS

Paresthesias may develop with peripheral nerve injuries or with central nervous system disease. They most commonly develop with metabolic neuropathy, such as that caused by diabetes mellitus or uremia. Patients with sarcoidosis, nutritional deficiencies, and traumatic nerve injuries also may complain of paresthesias.

### ANESTHESIA

With complete loss of sensation over any body surface, the skin becomes highly susceptible to injury. Patients with cervical syringomyelia often exhibit burns or perforating ulcers on their fingers if these become anesthetic as a consequence of the spinal cord damage. Denervation of deeper structures, such as joints, also causes damage to the largely anesthetic structure. The Charcot joint of tabes dorsalis is usually a damaged ankle joint that has lost pain sensation because of syphilitic damage to pain pathways. The most common cause of neuropathic anesthesia in the United States is diabetes mellitus. Pain perception may be lost superficially or deeply with this metabolic disease. Patients may develop foot ulcers from recurrent injuries to hypesthetic or anesthetic skin. Myocardial infarction may even occur without any associated pain in these individuals.

## SELECTED REFERENCES

Adams RD, Victor M: Principles of Neurology. 3rd ed. New York, McGraw-Hill, 1985.

Blumer D, Heilbronn M: Second-year follow up study on systematic treatment of chronic pain with antidepressants. Henry Ford Hosp Med J *29*:2, 1981.

Brown MJ, Asbury AK: Diabetic neuropathy. Ann Neurol *15*:2, 1984.

DeJong RH: Prof. Wall's three phases of pain. N Engl J Med *301*:1129, 1979.

Hendler N, Fernandez P: Alternative treatments for chronic pain. Psychiatr Ann *10*:495, 1980.

Fields HL: Pain II: New approaches to management. Ann Neurol *9*:101, 1981.

Fredericks JAM: Phantom limb and phantom limb pain. *In* Fredericks JAM (ed): Handbook of Clinical Neurology. Vol. 1: Clinical Neuropsychology. New York, Elsevier Science Publishers, 1985.

Kassirer MR, Osterberg DH: Pain in chronic multiple sclerosis. J Pain Sympt Manag *2*:95, 1987.

Portenoy RK (ed): Pain: Mechanisms and syndromes. Neurol Clin *7*:183, 1989.

Swerdlow M: Anticonvulsant drugs and chronic pain. Clin Neuropharmacol *7*:51, 1984.

Tomson T, Tybring G, Bertilsson L, et al: Carbamazepine therapy in trigeminal neuralgia. Arch Neurol *37*:699, 1980.

*Chapter 13*
# Headache and Facial Pain

Headaches may arise with disease in the head or neck. Facial pain usually reflects local disease or damage to the trigeminal nerve. The most commonly recognized headaches are from no apparent disease and are triggered by emotional stress. They are usually called tension headaches, but this name is not intended to dismiss the possibility that structural or chemical changes in or about the head are responsible for the pain.

## TENSION HEADACHE

Headaches triggered and sustained by emotional stress or conflict may be associated with musculoskeletal abnormalities. A normally asymptomatic degenerative arthritis of the neck may produce symptoms with stress. Painful cervical or masticatory muscle spasms may also develop with stress. Problems confused with tension headache include periodontal disease, temporomandibular joint dysfunction, dental malocclusion, eye strain, and cervical spine arthritis. The true tension headache usually has no consistent pattern. The patients' descriptions of the pain are often dramatic or fanciful. Women are more commonly affected than men. The patient with tension headache that has persisted more than a few weeks should be investigated with CT or MR scanning and EEG. Mild analgesics, such as aspirin or acetaminophen, are often sufficient to abort the headaches. Persistent headaches associated with no abnormalities evident on CT, MR, or EEG testing may require cerebrospinal fluid examination to eliminate the possibility of chronic meningitis.

## VASCULAR HEADACHE

A variety of vascular problems may cause headaches. The widely held notion that high blood pressure usually causes headaches is wrong, but extraordinary swings in blood pressure may cause transient headache. If intracranial hemorrhage is associated with the blood pressure problem, headache will be an acute problem. Vascular malformations occasionally are associated with recurrent headaches, even when no bleeding occurs. Unilateral eye pain, lid ptosis, and pupillary dilatation may develop with an enlarging aneurysm of the posterior communicating artery. Migraine and cluster headaches are from reversible vascular phenomena that are still poorly understood and are the types of vascular headaches most likely to recur chronically.

**Migraine**

Paroxysmal headaches developing primarily over one side of the head are usually migraine. These typically start between 15 and 22 years of age in both men and women and recur with variable frequency throughout young adult and middle-age life. With the most classic types of migraine, the patient has premonitory signs, called the aura, which may include evolving blindspots, focal weakness, or focal sensory complaints. The blindspots (scotomata) or visual field cuts may have distinctive scintillations or fortification patterns around them. Typically, the scotoma clears as the headache appears. The aura may last 20 to 30 minutes.

The pain of classic migraine usually lasts less than 3 hours. Nausea and vomiting often accompany the migraine pain. The pain is characteristically throbbing and also may be associated with diarrhea, polyuria, and diaphoresis. Most individuals with this headache prefer to remain inactive in a dark, quiet environment. Migraine attacks with some, but not all, of the facets of classic migraine are called common migraine. Women are much more susceptible to migraine headaches than are men.

Many different medications are used to manage migraine, but that most appropriate for the individual patient must be determined by the frequency, as well as the character, of the headache and the patient's overall health (Table 13-1). Ergotamine tartrate in combination with other medications is effective for many individuals and may be administered at the time the headache develops. Aspirin alone suffices to abort the migraine pain in a few patients, but acetaminophen combined with codeine or a mild barbiturate and caffeine is more typically effective. Methysergide was widely used for prevention of the headaches, but this drug is less widely used than it was decades ago because of cases of retroperitoneal fibrosis and fibrotic changes in heart valves reported with its use. Beta-blocking drugs, such as propranolol and metoprolol, have been effective when taken prophylactically, but the patient must have

TABLE 13-1.   *Medications for Migraine Attack*

| Medication | Dose | Frequency | Maximum |
|---|---|---|---|
| Aspirin 325 mg | 2 tab | every 4 to 6 hrs | 4 to 6 tabs daily |
| Aspirin + caffeine + butalbital (Fiorinal) | 1 tab | every 4 to 6 hrs | 4 to 6 tabs daily |
| Ergotamine tartrate 2 mg (Ergostat, Ergomar) | 1 tab | sublingual tab half-hourly | 3 tabs per day 5 tabs per week |
| Ergotamine tartrate + caffeine (Cafergot, Wigraine) | 1 tab | half-hourly during headache | 6 mg ergotamine per day 16 mg ergotamine per week |
| Acetaminophen 325 mg + codeine 15 mg (Tylenol #2) | 2 tab | every 4 to 6 hrs during headache | 4 to 6 tabs daily |

TABLE 13-2. *Migraine Prophylaxis*

| Medication | Dose | Frequency | Maximum |
|---|---|---|---|
| Propranolol hydrochloride 40 mg (Inderal) | 1 tab | 1 to 4 times daily | 4 to 8 tabs daily |
| Metoprolol tartrate 50 mg (Lopressor) | 1 tab | 1 to 4 times daily | 4 to 9 tabs daily |
| Amitriptyline hydrochloride 25 mg (Elavil) | 2 tab | 1 to 3 times daily | 2 to 6 daily |
| Methysergide maleate 2 mg (Sansert) | 1 tab | 2 to 4 times daily | 3 to 4 tabs daily |

migraine attacks more than once monthly to justify chronic use of these medications (Table 13-2). Other drugs with obvious efficacy include corticosteroids, such as prednisone, and phenothiazines, but these drugs have too many complications to make their use in the management of migraine reasonable.

### Cluster Headache

Cluster headache, or Horton histamine cephalgia or migrainous cranial neuralgia, presents as stabbing or boring pain in or about one eye with radiation to the side of the head ipsilateral to the painful eye. This type of vascular headache occurs most commonly in young or middle-aged men. The pain lasts 30 minutes to 2 hours and is associated with eyelid ptosis, pupillary miosis, conjunctival injection, nasal congestion, excessive tearing, and profound irritability. The affected individual is usually restless and combative. The headaches often occur in clusters over the course of a few weeks each year. Alcohol may trigger an attack. Some individuals have chronic cluster headache, with clusters lasting more than 4 months.

Drugs effective for individuals with cluster headache include methysergide and ergotamine tartrate. Ergotamine tartrate 2 mg taken before the attack may abort the headache. Some individuals are very sensitive to indomethacin taken daily or during the headaches. Others respond well to tricyclic antidepressant medications, such as imipramine or amitriptyline, or to lithium carbonate, 600 to 1200 mg daily. Phenothiazines, such as chlorpromazine, are usually effective against this type of headache, but the risks of acute dystonic reactions, tardive dyskinesias, and drug-induced parkinsonism make these drugs unacceptable options for treating this self-limited headache disorder.

Other considerations in patients with paroxysmal retro-orbital pain must include structural and inflammatory lesions behind the eye. If the patient has ocular motor problems and pupillary dilatation, as well as retro-orbital pain, an aneurysm in a posterior communicating artery may be responsible. Carotid-cavernous fistula, a pathologic connection between the internal carotid and the cavernous sinus, may cause similar problems. Painful ophthalmoplegia also develops with the Tolosa-Hunt syndrome, an idiopathic granulomatous disease of the cavernous sinus.

## Hypertensive Headache

Chronic high blood pressure is not an adequate explanation for chronic or paroxysmal headache, but diseases associated with hypertension may also be associated with headache. With profound hypertension, the patient may exhibit intracranial hemorrhage in association with seizures and altered consciousness, a condition usually called hypertensive encephalopathy and often preceded by severe headache. Patients receiving monoamine oxidase (MAO) inhibitors may develop acute hypertension and headache when exposed to tyramine-containing food. Such transient hypertension and headache may also develop with adrenal tumors, such as pheochromocytomas.

## Giant Cell Arteritis

Inflammatory disease of the cranial vasculature may produce severe headaches, especially in the elderly. The temporal and ophthalmic arteries are especially common sites of granulomatous disease, characterized by multinucleated giant cells in perivascular infiltrates. Patients with temporal artery involvement may complain of focal tenderness over the temples and pain on chewing. With ophthalmic artery involvement, acute visual loss may develop. Patients with giant cell arteritis also usually exhibit high erythrocyte sedimentation rates (ESR), low-grade fevers, weight loss, and malaise, as well as chronic headache. Temporal arteritis characteristically appears in individuals over 55 years of age who have an ESR of over 60 mm/hr. In many cases, the arteritis is sensitive to high-dose corticosteroid treatment.

## Vascular Malformation

Headache associated with vascular malformations may imitate migraine pain. What may help distinguish between the two are the persistence of focal deficits independent of the headache and the consistency with which the headache pain occurs on the same side of the head. Classically, migraine does not recur exclusively on one side of the head. Vascular malformations are prone to bleed with potentially fatal outcomes. The acute onset of severe headache during fornication, defecation, or pregnancy increases the probability that a vascular malformation is the underlying problem. Angiography will reveal the malformation unless it is the type designated cryptogenic, in which the primitive blood vessels are not perfused. Whenever possible, vascular malformations should be resected.

## POST-TRAUMATIC HEADACHE

Headache may occur chronically or episodically for years after a severe head injury. Acute post-traumatic headaches may actually be from the irritation caused by subarachnoid blood; chronic headaches raise the possibility of post-traumatic hydrocephalus. If the patient had CSF rhinorrhea or otorrhea associated with the trauma, headache developing within days or weeks of the injury may be the first sign of meningitis.

## INTRACRANIAL TUMORS

Brain tumors may cause headache, but they usually produce pain only late in their evolution. The headache that develops is usually from associated hydrocephalus or increased intracranial pressure. Tumors occasionally contact pain-sensitive structures, such as the inferior surface of the tentorium cerebelli, but more typically do not cause pain by direct impingement.

## PSEUDOTUMOR CEREBRI

Intracranial pressures greater than 200 or even 400 mm $H_2O$ may develop in children receiving vitamin supplements and in women with a variety of hormonal abnormalities or alterations, including those associated with pregnancy and obesity. The vitamin most often implicated is vitamin A. Some drugs, such as out-dated tetracycline and nalidixic acid, may be associated with the development of pseudotumor cerebri in some individuals.

The affected woman or child typically complains of persistent, diffuse, dull headache, occasionally associated with blurring of vision. Some of the affected individuals have vomiting and all have obvious papilledema. The clinical picture resembles that characteristic of a large intracranial mass; thus the name pseudotumor.

No hydrocephalus is associated with the increased intracranial pressure of pseudotumor cerebri, and herniation of the brain through the foramen magnum does not occur. Neuroimaging with CT or MR scanning reveals abnormally small ventricles. Visual field testing reveals an enlarged physiologic blindspot. Despite the unusual elevation of the cerebrospinal fluid pressure, the spinal fluid composition is normal.

Lumbar puncture may relieve the pressure for much longer than it ordinarily takes for the cerebrospinal fluid to be regenerated. The principal danger of pseudotumor cerebri is loss of vision from excessive pressure around the optic nerves. Some physicians recommend shunting the sheath around the optic nerves and also leaving a shunt in the intrathecal space to drain into the peritoneal cavity. More conservative measures include weight loss for women who are obese, provocative substance elimination for children who have had excessive exposure to vitamin A or antibiotics, and pregnancy termination for women who develop severe disease early in their pregnancies. High-dose corticosteroid treatment may reduce the intracranial pressure, but side effects of the steroids are usually counterproductive.

## CENTRAL NERVOUS SYSTEM INFECTION

Meningitis or meningoencephalitis may produce severe headache, neck stiffness, stupor, and seizures. It is atypical for a central nervous system infection to produce little more than headache and neck stiffness if it is not a self-limited problem. Fever, personality changes, and focal neurologic deficits or seizures routinely develop within hours or days of the appearance of more malignant infections. Notable exceptions include chronic tuberculous and cryptococcal meningitides. The patient's risk of meningitis, because of exposure or immunosuppression, must be taken into account. With chronic fungal or tuberculous meningitides, patients often develop cranial nerve deficits, such as facial nerve paralysis or ocular motor dysfunction, as the infection progresses. Lumbar puncture to evaluate cerebrospinal fluid parameters and to allow the fluid to be cultured is the investigation of choice whenever central nervous system infection is a probable cause of headache.

## SUBDURAL HEMATOMA

Chronic subdural hematomas may account for diffuse headaches appearing days or weeks after head trauma (Fig. 13-1). Patients at special risk for this intracranial mass include those on anticoagu-

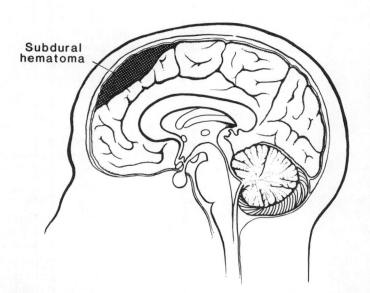

FIG. 13-1. Subdural hematomas may form over the convexity of the brain, as indicated in this schematic, and cause headache as one of their symptoms. (With permission from Lechtenberg R: Epilepsy and the Family. Cambridge, Harvard University Press, 1984.)

lants, those on hemodialysis, and those who are elderly. The sub-dural collection may produce little more than headache and de-mentia as it enlarges. It is a life-threatening problem because it may cause transtentorial or transfalcial herniation of the brain. MR or CT scanning usually reveals the subdural collection, but contrast enhancement may be necessary to define the mass on CT scanning. Chronic, as well as acute, subdural hematomas are surgical emer-gencies.

## INCREASED INTRACRANIAL PRESSURE

Headaches, either unilateral or bilateral, will develop with in-creased intracranial pressure arising for any reason. Hydrocephalus, an especially common cause of increased intracranial pressure, may be remedied with shunt placement. Hydrocephalus is usually de-scribed as communicating or noncommunicating, depending on whether the lateral ventricles communicate with the subarachnoid space. An obstruction at the aqueduct of Sylvius or at the foramina of Luschka or Magendie is the usual basis for obstructive hydro-cephalus. This type of obstruction may be relieved with ventricu-loperitoneal shunt placement.

## FACIAL PAIN

Designating facial pain as typical or atypical is largely of historical interest, but both terms are still used. Typical facial pain is sharp and short-lived with a distinct nidus of pain. Most patients with typical facial pain have trigeminal neuralgia. Atypical facial pain is more diffuse and chronic. Many of the patients affected have had recent facial or dental trauma. Any patient who has persistent facial pain, whether it is sharp or dull, must be evaluated for more ma-lignant causes of such discomfort, such as nasopharyngeal carcinoma or periodontal abscess.

### Tic Douloureux (Trigeminal Neuralgia)

With damage to the trigeminal nerve, patients may develop parox-ysmal facial pain triggered by specific stimuli or occurring sponta-neously. A specific stimulus to a limited area, such as touching a tooth or part of the gum, may trigger widespread pain. Because the trigger point is often in the mouth, many patients consult dentists first and have multiple tooth extractions. The pain of tic douloureux is usually limited to the second or third divisions of the trigeminal nerve, the maxillary and mandibular branches. Facial weakness does not typically occur along with the pain. If the facial pain is associated with a sixth nerve palsy, producing impaired abduction of the eye, the cause may be infectious petrositis. This association of facial pain, abducens nerve damage, and petrous pyramid osteomyelitis is Gra-denigo syndrome. Pain extending into the eye is unusual with tri-geminal neuralgia and should suggest a more malignant process, such as a retro-orbital tumor.

TABLE 13-3. *Drugs for Trigeminal Neuralgia*

| Drug | Brand | Dose | Frequency |
|------|-------|------|-----------|
| Carbamazepine | Tegretol | 200 mg | 3–6 times daily |
| Phenytoin | Dilantin | 100 mg | 3–4 times daily |
| Baclofen | Lioresal | 10 mg | 3–8 times daily |

Women suffer from trigeminal neuralgia three times as often as men. Individuals of either sex with many years of discomfort will still have preserved facial sensation. Many report that seasonal changes affect the pain, warm weather reducing the discomfort. What prompts the trigeminal nerve dysfunction is still unknown, but some evidence implicates a Herpes simplex infection. Some neurosurgeons have argued that vascular compression of the trigeminal nerve by the superior cerebellar or other large artery produces the pain.

Effective treatments include carbamazepine, phenytoin, and baclofen (Table 13-3). These oral medications must be used for weeks to eliminate and suppress the pain. Some patients do better on a combination of two drugs, but most who respond poorly to one drug will respond poorly to drug combinations. Which drug will be most effective is unpredictable. Most physicians use carbamazepine as their drug of choice, with phenytoin as their first alternative.

If medications fail, radiofrequency ablation of the trigeminal division or of the gasserian ganglion may be effective. The major complication of this and other surgical approaches is that the patient may be left with anesthesia dolorosa, a distracting wooden sensation associated with facial numbness. Operation on the posterior fossa performed to place cushioning material between the trigeminal nerve and overlying arteries has been successful in some individuals.

### Atypical Facial Pain

Atypical facial pain is less well localized and more constant a discomfort than tic douloureux. It may develop after facial trauma or dental work. In many cases, it has no apparent cause. There is no trigger point inciting the pain and no time of day when the pain is invariably worse. How important depression is in development of the pain has been argued for several decades. People with this chronic pain disorder are often depressed, and both the pain and the depression may clear with tricyclic antidepressant medication therapy. Imipramine given at 50 to 150 mg daily or amitriptyline at 25 to 75 mg daily are often highly effective in patients who can tolerate the drugs.

### Temporomandibular Joint Dysfunction

Malocclusion or local joint abnormalities may produce pain originating in or near the temporomandibular joint. This overdiagnosed joint disorder may be corrected with dental intervention, muscle relaxants, or in some cases antidepressants.

## Raeder Syndrome

Raeder syndrome is a facial pain disorder associated with granulomatous disease in the middle cranial fossa. A partial Horner syndrome accompanies the pain, miosis and lid ptosis being most evident. The cause of this disorder and its treatment are highly controversial. Malignancies or chronic meningitis should be sought whenever the syndrome is recognized.

## Postherpetic Neuralgia

Pain may develop after Herpes zoster infections. Characteristic vesicles appear along the distribution of the affected nerve. Most infections are presumed to be reactivations of long dormant viruses, because most individuals acquire the virus during childhood but develop the acute radicular disease, colloquially known as shingles, late in adult life.

Although post-herpetic neuralgia may develop anywhere on the body, the part of the face supplied by the ophthalmic division of the trigeminal nerve is most likely to be affected when the virus causes an eruption on the face. Acute care of the inflammatory lesion requires ophthalmologic measures that are best managed by a specialist. Tricyclic antidepressants or carbamazepine may help to suppress the chronic pain that often develops in the distribution of the sensory nerves injured by the virus.

## SELECTED REFERENCES

Albers GW, Simon LT, Hamik A, et al: Nifedipine versus propranolol for the initial prophylaxis of migraine. Headache *29*:215, 1989.

Blier P, DeMontigny C, Chaput Y: Modifications of the serotonin system by antidepressant treatments. J Clin Psychopharmacol *7*(Suppl 6):24S, 1987.

Brisman R: Trigeminal neuralgia and multiple sclerosis. Arch Neurol *44*:379, 1987.

Burchiel KJ, Clarke H, Haglund M, et al: Longterm efficacy of microvascular decompression in trigeminal neuralgia. J Neurosurg *69*:35, 1988.

Caviness VS Jr, O'Brien P: Current concepts: Headache. N Engl J Med *302*:446, 1980.

Diamond S, Dalessio DJ: The Practicing Physician's Approach to Headache. 4th Ed. Baltimore, Williams & Wilkins, 1986.

Friedman AP: Headache. *In* Baker AB, Baker LH (eds): Clinical Neurology. Philadelphia, Harper and Row, 1986, pp 1–50.

Heyck H: Pathogenesis of migraine. Res Clin Stud Headache *2*:1, 1989.

Kudrow L: Cluster headache: Diagnosis and management. Headache *19*:142, 1979.

Lance JW: Headache. Neurology *10*:1, 1981.

Lance JW: Fifty years of migraine research. Aust NZ J Med *18*:311, 1988.

Lance JW: A concept of migraine and the search for the ideal headache drug. Headache *30* (Suppl 1):17, 1990.

Peatfield RC, Fozard JR, Rose FC: Drug treatment of migraine. *In* Rose FC (ed): Handbook of Clinical Neurology. Vol. 4. New York, Elsevier, 1986, p 173.

Peroutka SJ: The pharmacology of current anti-migraine drugs. Headache *30* (Suppl 1):5, 1990.

Portenoy RK (ed): Pain: Mechanisms and syndromes. Neurologic Clinics *7*:183, 1989.

Raskin NH, Schwartz RK: Icepick-like pain. Neurology *30:*203, 1980.
Raskin NH, Hosobuchi Y, Lamb S: Headache may arise from perturbation of brain. Headache *27:*416, 1987.
Saper JR: Drug treatment of headache: Changing concepts and treatment strategies. Semin Neurol *7:*178, 1987.

# Chapter 14

# Disturbed Vision

Many diseases cause transient or permanent loss of vision. The most common causes of visual loss in the United States are glaucoma and diabetes mellitus. Both of these impair vision by damaging the retina and are usually easily diagnosed before retinal damage has progressed to complete visual loss. Intraocular pressures may be reduced by drug treatment or ocular surgery in the patient with glaucoma, and retinopathy may be slowed in patients with diabetes by laser surgery on the retina.

## AMAUROSIS FUGAX

Amaurosis fugax is a transient loss of vision in one eye. It occurs most often as a result of vascular disease in or small emboli to the eye affected (Table 14-1). Platelet or cholesterol emboli may transiently obstruct a large branch of the ophthalmic artery and then break up. With disintegration of the embolus, the patient may recover vision. If an obstruction persists for more than a few minutes, ischemic damage to the retina will be permanent. Irreversible ischemic damage to the optic nerve is called ischemic optic neuropathy.

In younger adults, amaurosis fugax is rarely followed by a stroke. The vascular disease in these individuals is probably inflammatory, rather than obstructive. Spasm of the ophthalmic artery occurs with some types of headaches, including cluster headaches, so transient loss of vision in these young individuals may be a result of completely reversible ischemic episodes.

## OPTIC NEURITIS

Optic neuritis, inflammatory disease of an optic nerve, may also produce transient visual loss in one eye, but most causes of optic neuritis leave the patient with residual deficits. Multiple sclerosis is a relatively common cause of optic neuritis in young adults. With multiple sclerosis, demyelination of nerve fibers occurs in the optic nerve or tract, much of that demyelination persisting even after the patient has a remission of symptoms. The optic neuritis may be painful, and if the inflammation is close enough to the optic disc, the patient may appear to have papilledema. This inflammatory change of the optic disc is more appropriately called papillitis. If the inflammation is much closer to the optic chiasm, the patient may have no apparent changes in the disc despite the development of monocular blindness. This is retrobulbar neuritis, a common cause of transient monocular blindness. Steroids reduce the pain of optic neuritis associated with multiple sclerosis, but have little or

TABLE 14-1. *Causes of Transient Visual Loss*

| Visual Field Cut | Blindness In One Eye | Complete Blindness |
|---|---|---|
| Transient ischemia | Optic neuritis | Bilateral optic neuritis |
| Migraine | Transient ischemia | Vertebrobasilar insufficiency |
| Focal sensory seizures | Trauma to the eye | Basilar impression |
| Optic chiasm compression | Optic nerve compression | |
| Glaucoma | | |

no effect on the extent of visual impairment that persists after the acute flareup remits.

## OPTIC ATROPHY

After the inflammation of optic neuritis has abated, the optic disc has decreased vasculature and a chalky appearance characteristic of optic atrophy. Many infections, such as histoplasmosis, also can cause optic neuritis with subsequent optic atrophy. Even neuro-syphilis may cause optic atrophy as a late manifestation of CNS involvement by the spirochete. Patients with optic atrophy exhibit the Marcus-Gunn afferent pupillary defect and have abnormal visual evoked potentials (Fig. 14-1).

Tumors impinging on an optic nerve may produce transient episodes of visual loss associated with slowly evolving optic atrophy. A meningioma on the sphenoid bone is the most common cause of this problem. The increased intracranial pressure associated with the tumor will produce papilledema in the uncompressed optic nerve. Papilledema with contralateral optic atrophy associated with a meningioma impinging on the atrophic optic nerve is called the Foster-Kennedy syndrome.

## TRANSIENT BINOCULAR BLINDNESS

Transient blindness in both eyes occurs much less frequently than does amaurosis fugax, but it too may develop with optic neuritis. Obviously, significant inflammatory disease in both optic nerves must occur to produce bilateral blindness. Ischemia to the occipital lobes with vertebrobasilar disease may also produce reversible blindness. This occasionally appears with basilar migraine, vertebrobasilar insufficiency, and basilar impression. A tumor overlying the occipital lobes may produce transient visual field defects, transient binocular blindness, or visual hallucinations. These tumor-induced alterations in vision arise from compression of blood vessels supplying the occipital lobes or from direct irritation of the occipital lobe cortex (Fig. 14-2).

## VISUAL FIELD DEFECTS

The physiologic blindspot created by the optic nerve at the point it originates on the retina is called the cecal scotoma. Blindspots

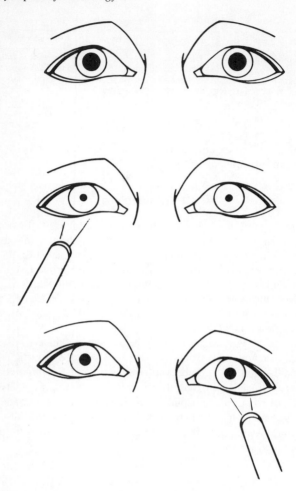

FIG. 14-1. The Marcus-Gunn afferent pupillary defect is characterized by equally dilated pupils in normal lighting. With light shined into the normal eye, both pupils constrict. On swinging the flashlight to the eye with the afferent defect, both pupils appear to dilate paradoxically. (With permission from Lechtenberg R: Multiple Sclerosis Fact Book. Philadelphia, F.A. Davis, 1988.)

involving central vision are central scotomata. If a blindspot originates in central vision and extends to the cecal blindspot or the cecal blindspot enlarges adequately to impinge on central vision, the resulting visual field defect is called a centrocecal scotoma (Fig. 14-3). Centrocecal scotomata are seen most often with $B_{12}$ and other vitamin deficiencies, alcohol or tobacco abuse, retinal histoplasmosis, and pseudotumor cerebri.

Transient visual field defects develop routinely with classic migraine. Vertebrobasilar insufficiency may produce a transient field cut, but more often, it produces complete blindness. Glaucoma may produce transient scotomata, but with recurrent damage to the ret-

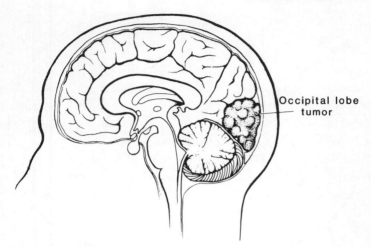

Occipital lobe
tumor

FIG. 14-2. Occipital lobe tumors, as indicated in this schematic, may cause sufficient compression of the blood vessels supplying the visual cortex to produce visual field defects. (With permission from Lechtenberg R: Epilepsy And the Family. Cambridge, Harvard University Press, 1984.)

ina, the patient usually develops persistent scotomata. The blind-spots associated with retinal damage from glaucoma are usually sickle-shaped. Long-standing glaucoma may even produce a characteristic binasal hemianopia.

One of the more easily recognized field defects is the bitemporal hemianopia that develops with compression of the optic chiasm (Table 14-2). Pituitary masses impinging on the chiasm from below routinely produce this type of defect, but the defect is fixed rather than transient.

Visual defects may develop with damage to the retina, optic nerve, chiasm, optic tract, lateral geniculate, optic radiation, or occipital cortex. The more posterior in the visual system is the defect, the more symmetric are the field defects evident in each eye.

## CORTICAL BLINDNESS

Bilateral occipital lobe injuries may produce blindness. Patients with complete cortical blindness may have visual confabulations: they report seeing highly detailed scenes and deny their blindness. The combination of cortical blindness and visual confabulation is called Anton syndrome. This is different from visual agnosia or psychic blindness, in which the patient has no loss of vision and yet cannot recognize items he sees.

## DIPLOPIA

The acute appearance of double vision or diplopia usually indicates an acute ocular motor problem (Table 14-3). The underlying

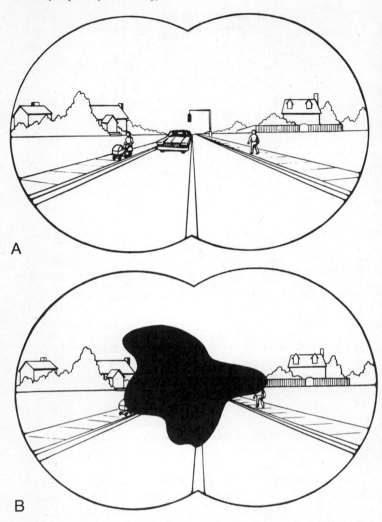

FIG. 14-3. Instead of high acuity in the center of the field of vision (A), the patient with a centrocecal scotoma has impaired central vision but preserved peripheral vision (B). (With permission from Lechtenberg R: Multiple Sclerosis Fact Book. Philadelphia, F.A. Davis, 1988.)

TABLE 14-2.  *Field Defects*

| Type | Pattern | Common Causes |
|------|---------|---------------|
| Homonymous hemianopia | Half of field defective on same side in both eyes | Stroke<br>Brain tumor<br>Brain abscess |
| Bitemporal hemianopia | Lateral half of visual field defective in both eyes | Mass on optic chiasm |
| Binasal hemianopia | Medial half of visual field defective in both eyes | Glaucoma |
| Homonymous quadrantanopia | One quarter of visual field lost on same side in both eyes | Temporal or parietal lesion |

TABLE 14-3.  *Causes of Diplopia*

Hysteria
Trauma
Diabetes mellitus
Brainstem infarction
Myasthenia gravis
Thyroid disease
Multiple sclerosis
Posterior fossa tumors
Drug effects
Meningeal carcinomatosis
Meningitis
Nasopharyngeal carcinoma
Intraorbital masses
Posterior inferior communicating artery aneurysm
Increased intracranial pressure

disease is suggested by the patient's age and other medical problems. An elderly patient who also has hypertension must be presumed to have had a brainstem stroke until proven otherwise. Young patients with diabetes mellitus are at risk for infarction of the oculomotor nerve.

Other diseases commonly causing diplopia include myasthenia gravis, meningeal carcinomatosis, and posterior fossa tumors. Trauma to the orbit may disturb ocular motor function sufficiently to pro-

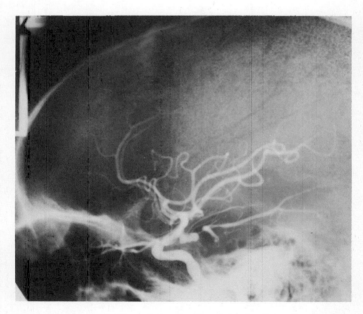

FIG. 14-4. This angiogram of the vessels originating from the internal carotid artery reveals a lobulated aneurysm on the otherwise thin posterior communicating artery. This aneurysm invariably impinges on the oculomotor nerve and produces mydriasis, ptosis, and disturbed activity of the medial rectus, inferior rectus, superior rectus, and inferior oblique muscles. (From Lechtenberg R: The Psychiatrist's Guide to Diseases of the Nervous System. New York, John Wiley and Sons, 1982.)

duce double vision, a complication that may develop even if no fracture of the orbit occurred. Increased intracranial pressure may produce an abducens nerve (cranial nerve VI) dysfunction, with resultant lateral rectus weakness. An aneurysm on the posterior communicating artery usually impinges on the oculomotor (cranial nerve III) and produces medial rectus, superior rectus, inferior rectus, and inferior oblique weakness (Fig. 14-4). Involvement of these cranial nerves produces diplopia, which is most evident when the patient attempts to look in directions that require contraction of the weak muscles.

## SELECTED REFERENCES

Miller DH, Ormerod IEC, McDonald WI, et al: The early risk of multiple sclerosis after optic neuritis. J Neurol Neurosurg Psychiatry *51*:1569, 1988.
Tippin J. Corbett JJ, Kerber, RE, et al: Amaurosis fugax and ocular infarction in adolescents and young adults. Ann Neurol *26*:69, 1989.

# Chapter 15
# Vertigo, Dizziness, and Hearing Disturbances

Diseases of the ear and of the nerves originating in the ear often produce dizziness, vertigo, hearing loss, or combinations of these complaints. The proximity of the cochlea and the semicircular canals, as well as that of the acoustic and vestibular components of the auditory cranial nerve (VIII), makes damage to the balance system a common feature of damage to the hearing apparatus.

## DIZZINESS AND VERTIGO

Dizziness is a subjective complaint of postural instability. Vertigo is the actual perception of illusory environmental rotation. Nausea and vomiting commonly accompany vertigo. Standing may be difficult with dizziness, but it becomes virtually impossible with vertigo. Either of these complaints may develop with brainstem, cerebellar, or inner ear disease.

### Labyrinthitis

Inflammatory disease of the labyrinth or of the vestibular division of the eighth cranial nerve is usually referred to as labyrinthitis or vestibular neuronitis. These inflammatory disorders routinely produce vertigo and may produce hearing loss as well. In most cases, they are presumed to be caused by viruses and are self-limited. If episodes of vertigo occur repeatedly, are unassociated with any progressive lesions, and have symptoms that are worsened by positional changes, the clinical picture is usually called benign recurrent or benign positional vertigo.

### Vertebrobasilar Insufficiency

Insufficient blood flow through the vertebrobasilar system is also a common cause of transient dizziness or vertigo. Narrowing or obstruction of the vertebral arteries is the usual basis for this insufficiency, but occasionally a reversal of flow patterns, such as that occurring with subclavian steal, is responsible for the brainstem signs and symptoms that develop. Alternative causes to be considered with signs of vertebrobasilar insufficiency include cerebellopontine angle tumors and posterior fossa meningiomas.

### Posterior Fossa Tumors

Tumors in the posterior fossa that compress the cerebellum or cranial nerve VIII may cause vertigo. Schwannomas of the

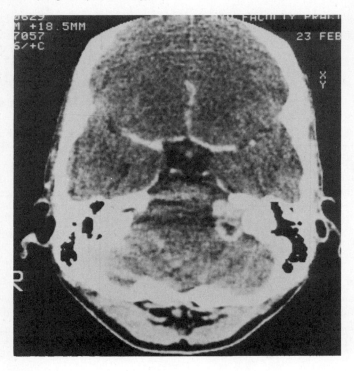

FIG. 15-1. A small schwannoma is apparent at the internal auditory meatus on this CT scan through the petrous pyramids. (With permission from Lechtenberg R: Seizure Recognition and Treatment. New York, Churchill Livingstone, 1989.)

vestibular division of the auditory nerve commonly arise in neurofibromatosis, but may occur independently of this hereditary disorder (Fig. 15-1). Meningiomas may also arise near enough to the cerebellopontine angle to cause auditory nerve compression. Medulloblastomas, ependymomas, and astrocytomas of the cerebellum often produce vertigo through direct injury to the cerebellum or the brainstem.

## HEARING DISTURBANCES

Hearing loss usually develops with damage to the ear or acoustic nerve. Very loud noises cause acoustic trauma, a cochlear injury that may result in permanent hearing loss. Degenerative cochlear disease, recurrent otitis media, and otosclerosis are more slowly progressive causes of hearing loss.

Some hearing impairment may occur with demyelination in the brainstem, such as in multiple sclerosis, with vertebrobasilar insufficiency, such as in a subclavian steal syndrome, or with malignant tumors, such as meningeal carcinomatosis. In most instances in which damage to the brainstem provides the basis for impaired hearing, other cranial nerve signs are also evident. Deafness is highly improbable on the basis of brainstem disease alone.

Deafness does not occur with strictly cortical lesions, even if the lesions are bilateral. Hearing may be disturbed with temporal lobe lesions, but receptive aphasia is much more likely than impaired auditory acuity. Damage to the right cerebral hemisphere may disturb musical recognition in people who are not trained musicians.

## Auditory Agnosia

Problems with auditory recognition are generally grouped together as the auditory agnosias. Patients may be unable to recognize specific types of noise, even when they have preserved language comprehension, pure-tone audiometry, and speech recognition.

## Auditory Hallucinations

Auditory hallucinations in young people suggest drug abuse, schizophrenia, or complex partial seizures. With delirium tremens, the alcoholic individual may have extremely vivid and threatening visual or auditory hallucinations, but the hallucinations are closely linked to alcohol withdrawal and are not easily confused with persistent cognitive disorders. In some cases, auditory hallucinations develop with chronic meningoencephalitis or a subarachnoid hemorrhage.

## Tinnitus

The perception of ringing or whistling noises independent of external stimuli is called tinnitus. Many individuals with hearing loss have tinnitus. Patients often believe that it is the illusory noise, rather than ear damage, that is interfering with their hearing.

Tinnitus is a major component of Meniere syndrome, an auditory syndrome in which hearing loss is associated with episodes of vertigo and transient or persistent tinnitus. Many patients develop Meniere syndrome as part of endolymphatic hydrops, a disturbance of cochlear and vestibular fluid regulation.

The most common causes of persistent tinnitus are acoustic trauma and drug effects (Table 15-1). Aspirin is the drug most often implicated in tinnitus, but a wide variety of medications may induce this hearing disturbance as a side effect. Schwannomas of cranial nerve VIII may present with tinnitus, but this is an unusual cause of a common symptom.

TABLE 15-1.  *Causes of Tinnitus*

| |
| --- |
| Acoustic trauma |
| Meniere syndrome |
| Drug effect |
| Posterior fossa tumor |
| Arteriovenous malformation |
| Brainstem injury |

Tinnitus may be suppressed with some benzodiazepines, such as clonazepam (Klonopin) and lorazepam (Ativan), but the sedative effects of these drugs limit their applicability. Devices producing sounds that mask the tinnitus may be more effective and practical for many of the patients with this complaint.

## SELECTED REFERENCES

Asbury, AK, McKhann GM, McDonald WI (eds): Diseases of the Nervous System. Clinical Neurobiology. Philadelphia, W.B. Saunders, 1986.

Baloh RW, Honrubia V: Clinical Neurophysiology of the Vestibular System. Philadelphia, F.A. Davis, 1979.

Barber HO: Current ideas on vestibular diagnosis. Otolaryngol Clin North Am *11*:283, 1978.

Brandt T, Daroff RB: The multisensory physiology and pathological vertigo syndromes. Ann Neurol 7:195, 1980.

Goodhill V (ed): Ear Diseases, Deafness, and Dizziness. New York, Harper and Row, 1979.

Huson SM, Harper PS, Compston DAS: Von Recklinghausen neurofibromatosis. A clinical and population study in southeast Wales. Brain *111*:1355, 1988.

Rowland LP (ed): Merritt's Textbook of Neurology. 8th Ed. Philadelphia, Lea & Febiger, 1989.

# Chapter 16
# Stroke

Stroke is an irreversible ischemic or hemorrhagic injury to CNS tissue. Patients with strokes may recover completely from their deficits, but most individuals with vascular injuries of the brain will have residual signs or symptoms. Stroke may occur with venous disease, such as venous or sinus thrombosis, but much less commonly than with arterial occlusion or hemorrhage (Fig. 16-1). Atherosclerosis and chronic hypertension are the most common causes of stroke, but other problems may be responsible. Valvular heart disease may release emboli that obstruct cerebral vessels. An often overlooked basis for cerebrovascular accidents is infection. Some infections, such as those associated with syphilis (Heubner's arteritis, Nissl's arteritis) or Lyme disease (neuroborreliosis), may cause occlusive vasculitis.

Not all strokes are symptomatic. About 10% of stroke patients have MRI or CT evidence of preexisting silent strokes. Most of the individuals with silent strokes have diabetes mellitus or abnormal glucose tolerance tests.

Stroke itself may prove lethal if massive edema or extensive bleeding in the head associated with the stroke cause herniation of the brain across the falx cerebri, tentorium cerebelli, or foramen magnum. Most patients with strokes, however, die from cardiovascular disease, rather than from the brain injury.

## INFARCTION

When ischemia lasts several minutes, infarction of brain tissue occurs. Most ischemia develops with vascular occlusion from local or remote disease. In the brain, local lesions include intimal hyperplasia associated with chronic hypertension, vasospasm associated with subarachnoid hemorrhage, or atherosclerosis associated with hypercholesterolemia. Emboli from atheromatous plaques outside the brain may travel into the internal carotid or vertebral arteries and produce occlusion. Diseased heart valves also routinely produce emboli to the head. The most common settings for this valvular heart disease include rheumatic fever, bacterial endocarditis, and systemic lupus erythematosus.

Individuals who have had transient ischemic attacks (TIAs) are at an increased risk of having a stroke, but most strokes that occur after a TIA occur during the first few weeks. The risk of ischemic stroke is significantly increased in individuals who smoke or have hypertension, diabetes mellitus, or hyperlipidemia. Ischemic strokes occurring in individuals under 50 years of age should not be ascribed to chronic hypertension or uncomplicated atherosclerosis. Hyper-

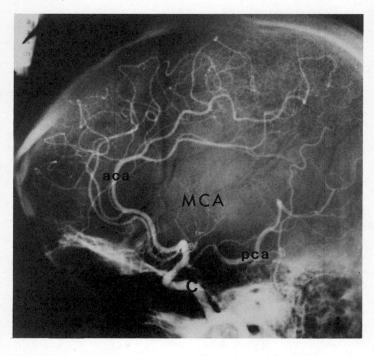

FIG. 16-1. This patient developed complete occlusion of the middle cerebral artery. The cortex (MCA) supplied by this artery was infarcted, but that supplied by the anterior cerebral artery (aca) and posterior cerebral artery (pca) were unaffected (C = internal carotid artery). (From Lechtenberg R: The Psychiatrist's Guide to Diseases of the Nervous System. New York, John Wiley and Sons, 1982.)

lipidemia, hemoglobinopathies (e.g., sickle cell disease), coagulation defects, valvular heart disease, and other causes of vascular occlusion must be sought.

The risk of death with nonhemorrhagic stroke in men is directly proportional to the total serum cholesterol level, but most of these men dying within a few years after a stroke succumb to cardiovascular disease.

### Common Carotid Artery Occlusion

More than 80% of patients who develop common carotid artery occlusion have TIAs. If the common carotid is occluded, the patient need not exhibit any persistent neurologic deficits. Collaterals to the internal carotid and other vessels supplying the brain often fully compensate for occlusions of the common carotid. Individuals who do have symptomatic occlusions are usually women with a history of smoking, hypertension, diabetes mellitus, hyperlipidemia, or a combination of these risk factors. Signs and symptoms of an occlusion are diverse and include visual problems, weakness, sensory

TABLE 16-1. *Syndromes Associated with Major Vessel Occlusions*

| Artery | Deficits |
|--------|----------|
| Left middle cerebral | Right-sided weakness, arm and face more than leg <br> Right-sided sensory loss <br> Expressive aphasia, usually <br> Global aphasia, occasionally <br> Left gaze preference, at least transiently <br> Right homonymous hemianopia, partial or total |
| Right anterior cerebral | Left-sided weakness, leg more than arm or face <br> Left-sided sensory loss, primarily in leg <br> Urinary incontinence, often <br> Affective disorder, commonly |
| Left posterior cerebral | Right-sided homonymous hemianopia <br> Impaired reading, usually <br> Impaired memory <br> Brainstem signs, variably |
| Posterior inferior cerebellar (PICA) (Wallenberg syndrome) | Ipsilateral limb ataxia and hypotonia <br> Impaired ipsilateral facial sensation <br> Impaired ipsilateral corneal reflex <br> Impaired contralateral limb and trunk pain perception <br> Ipsilateral Horner syndrome <br> Gait ataxia <br> Nausea and vomiting <br> Nystagmus <br> Dysarthria <br> Dysphagia |
| Anterior inferior cerebellar (AICA) | Ipsilateral limb ataxia <br> Ipsilateral Horner syndrome <br> Ipsilateral deafness <br> Ipsilateral facial weakness <br> Impaired corneal reflex <br> Impaired ipsilateral facial pain perception <br> Impaired contralateral limb and trunk pain perception <br> Vertigo <br> Dysarthria <br> Nystagmus <br> Nausea and vomiting |
| Superior cerebellar | Ipsilateral limb dysmetria <br> Ipsilateral Horner syndrome <br> Impaired contralateral pain and temperature perception <br> Impaired hearing |

disturbances, dysarthria, tremors, headache, lightheadedness, and syncope (Table 16-1).

## Vertebrobasilar System

Occlusion of the basilar artery is often fatal, but obstruction of an individual vertebral artery is not likely to have substantial consequences if the other vertebral artery is patent and none of the major branches of the vertebral artery is occluded. Branches of the vertebral artery that produce characteristic syndromes when occluded include the posterior inferior cerebellar artery (PICA), anterior inferior cerebellar artery (AICA), and the superior cerebellar artery (SCA).

TABLE 16-2. *Causes of Stroke in Young People*

| Disorder | Examples |
|---|---|
| Endocarditis | Subacute bacterial endocarditis |
| | Libman-Sacks (lupus) endocarditis |
| Hypercoagulable states | Hormone-induced |
| | Pregnancy-associated |
| Vascular spasm | Complicated migraine |
| Vascular malformation | Arteriovenous malformation |
| | Aneurysm |
| Hemoglobinopathy | Sickle cell disease |

## HEMIPARESIS

Unilateral weakness occurs with many different types of stroke. With chronic hypertension, pure motor strokes producing weakness alone are relatively common. The patient usually develops substantial weakness or paralysis (hemiplegia) of one side of the body over the course of minutes or hours. The site of disease is usually the contralateral internal capsule or pons. Damage to the crus cerebri may also produce hemiparesis, but this type of midbrain lesion is considerably less common than pontine or capsular lesions. The midbrain lesion is also likely to be associated with an ocular motor problem because of damage to the third cranial nerve or its nucleus.

Young adults may develop hemiparesis as a consequence of vasculitis or valvular heart disease (Table 16-2). The young person with aortic or mitral valve damage from rheumatic fever or intravenous drug abuse is at high risk of emboli to the brain. Young women with systemic lupus erythematosus may exhibit hemiparesis associated with a lupus vasculitis of the cerebral vasculature. Systemic lupus also produces valvular heart disease in some individuals, a complication called Libman-Sacks endocarditis, thereby placing those individuals at risk of suffering embolic damage to the brain. Some hematologic disorders, such as sickle cell anemia, may cause infarction without any embolic events if blood flow through the cerebral vasculature is disrupted by changes in the blood cells. Blood viscosity may also increase and interfere with cerebral perfusion in neoplasias producing paraproteinemia.

## INTRACEREBRAL HEMORRHAGE

Spontaneous intracerebral hemorrhage most often develops in chronic hypertension. Favored sites for these hemorrhages include the caudate, putamen, thalamus, pons, and cerebellum. Bleeding originates primarily in microscopic aneurysmal defects in blood vessel walls. These Charcot-Bouchard aneurysms may cause lethal hemorrhages when they bleed and are not treatable before they self-destruct.

Hemorrhages may develop in individuals with clotting disorders for no apparent reason, but in most cases head trauma is associated with the bleeding. Some poorly understood vasculopathies are also associated with intracerebral hemorrhages. Cerebral amyloid or congophilic angiopathy is one such disorder. Patients who develop this angiopathy usually have significant atherosclerotic disease in the circle of Willis and elsewhere in the body. Hemorrhages in amyloid angiopathy occur outside the locations typical for hemorrhages associated with hypertension. Several small, nonlethal hemorrhages may occur in affected individuals.

## SUBARACHNOID HEMORRHAGE

Subarachnoid hemorrhage may occur as the extension of an intracerebral hemorrhage or independently. Patients with this type of bleeding usually complain of headache, photophobia, nausea, and vomiting. Seizures may develop; and even if seizures do not occur, confusion or coma is likely.

Causes of bleeding into the subarachnoid space include head trauma, aneurysmal bleeds, coagulation defects, and angiopathies, such as that associated with systemic lupus erythematosus. The blood in the subarachnoid space may cause focal neurologic deficits or seizures. The focal deficits are presumed to occur as a consequence of ischemia triggered by the presence of subarachnoid blood. Intracranial vessels irritated by the blood are likely to develop spasm and therefore carry less blood to brain tissues.

Much of the management of subarachnoid hemorrhage has involved efforts to reduce the vascular spasm and attendant ischemia that usually develop. Nimodipine administered at 60 mg 4 times daily for 3 weeks is the only drug with established efficacy in reducing the probability of ischemia associated with subarachnoid hemorrhage.

The chemical meningitis induced by subarachnoid hemorrhage may produce hydrocephalus. Presumably, inflammatory changes along the meninges interfere with CSF reabsorption. Patients who develop hydrocephalus after a subarachnoid hemorrhage have a poorer prognosis than those who do not.

## ANEURYSMS

Defects in the walls of arteries may allow outpouchings or aneurysms to form. These may be called saccular or fusiform, depending on whether they have a neck. Specific diseases may produce specific types of aneurysms. With subacute bacterial endocarditis, patients may develop small aneurysms on the superficial vessels over the convexities of the hemispheres. These are called mycotic aneurysms. If they bleed, it is usually into the subarachnoid space. With chronic hypertension, patients may develop microscopic aneurysms on the vessels supplying diencephalic structures, such as the basal ganglia and the thalamus. These are called Charcot-Bouchard aneurysms, and when they bleed, it is usually into the brain parenchyma.

Large saccular aneurysms in adults usually develop in or near the

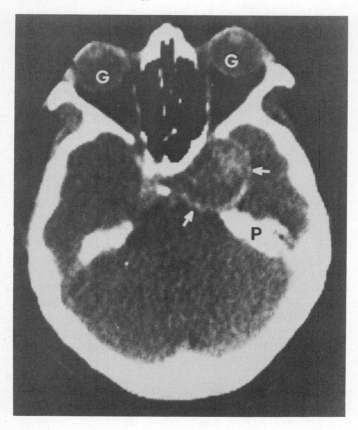

FIG. 16-2. Giant aneurysms in the circle of Willis (arrows) may produce chiasmatic compression and imitate tumors in the suprasellar region (P = petrous pyramid; G = globe of eye). (From Lechtenberg R: The Psychiatrist's Guide to Diseases of the Nervous System. New York, John Wiley and Sons, 1982.)

elements of the circle of Willis (Fig. 16-2). The bifurcation of the internal carotid and middle cerebral artery is an especially common site for a symptomatic saccular aneurysm. The anterior and posterior communicating arteries are also relatively common sites for saccular aneurysms. Bleeding from any of these aneurysms usually produces subarachnoid blood as well as intraparenchymal blood. The posterior communicating artery (PCA) aneurysm is often symptomatic before bleeding occurs because of its proximity to the oculomotor nerve. Patients complain of headache and blurred or double vision and exhibit oculomotor paresis, ptosis, and mydriasis.

Aneurysms are relatively uncommon in the posterior fossa. When they do occur, they are usually at the bifurcation of the basilar artery into the posterior cerebral arteries. Bleeding from a saccular aneurysm in this location usually produces an abrupt loss of consciousness.

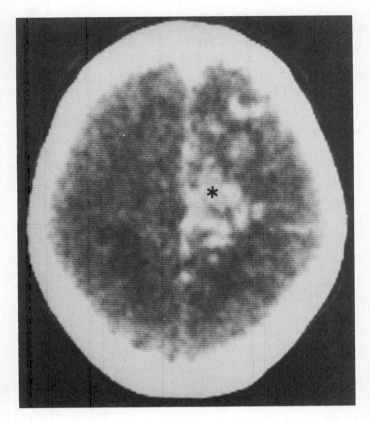

FIG. 16-3. The postcontrast CT scan may reveal the serpiginous vessels of large arteriovenous malformations (*). (With permission from Lechtenberg R: Seizure Recognition and Treatment. New York, Churchill Livingstone, 1990.)

## ARTERIOVENOUS MALFORMATIONS

Congenital vascular malformations change with age and often bleed. Even if a lethal or disabling hemorrhage does not develop, the abnormal blood vessels may enlarge enough to impair the function of nearby brain or spinal cord tissue. Otherwise asymptomatic malformations may irritate nearby cerebral cortex and produce seizures (Fig. 16-3). The lesions may be diagnosed with MR or CT scanning, but the extent of the vascular malformation usually cannot be established without angiography. Large malformations may be unresectable without presurgical obstruction of some constituent vessels. This obstruction is usually accomplished by using a silicon glue or spheres introduced into the malformation during angiography. Complete resection of the abnormal system of vessels is preferrable but is not always feasible. The vessels supplying the vascular malformation may also be supplying vital structures in the brain or spinal cord.

## SELECTED REFERENCES

Barnett HJM, Mohr JP, Stein BM, Yatsu FM (eds): Stroke. Pathophysiology, Diagnosis, and Management. New York, Churchill Livingstone, 1986.

Ferreiro JA, Ansbacher LE, Vinters HV: Stroke related to cerebral amyloid angiopathy: The significance of systemic vascular disease. J Neurol *236*:267, 1989.

Gilman S, Bloedel J, Lechtenberg R: Disorders of the cerebellum. Philadelphia, F.A. Davis, 1981.

Gorelick PB, Rodin MB, Langenberg P, et al: Weekly alcohol consumption, cigarette smoking, and the risk of ischemic stroke: Results of a case-control study at three urban medical centers in Chicago, Illinois. Neurology *39*:339, 1989.

Graff-Radford NR, Torner J, Adams HP Jr, Kassell NF: Factors associated with hydrocephalus after subarachnoid hemorrhage. A report of the Cooperative Aneurysm Study. Arch Neurol *46*:744, 1989.

Iso H, Jacobs DR, Jr, Wentworth D, et al: Serum cholesterol levels and six-year mortality from stroke in 350,977 men screened for multiple risk factor intervention trial. N Engl J Med *320*:904, 1989.

Kase CS, Wolf PA, Chodosh EH, et al: Prevalence of silent stroke in patients presenting with initial stroke: The Framingham study. Stroke *20*:850, 1989.

Levine SR, Welch KMA: Common carotid artery occlusion. Neurology *39*:178, 1989.

Pickard JD, Murray GD, Illingworth R, et al: Effect of oral nimodipine on cerebral infarction and outcome after subarachnoid hemorrhage: British aneurysm nimodipine trial. Br Med J *298*:636, 1989.

Prohovnik I, Pavlakis SG, Piomelli S, et al: Cerebral hyperemia, stroke, and transfusion in sickle cell disease. Neurology *39*:344, 1989.

Tippin J. Corbett JJ, Kerber RE, et al: Amaurosis fugax and ocular infarction in adolescents and young adults. Ann Neurol *26*:69, 1989.

# Chapter 17
# Neoplastic Disease

Primary brain tumors, that is, those arising in the brain, account for about 2 to 5% of all tumors. They are the most common solid tumors occurring during childhood. Although controversy surrounds the cells of origin of some of the primary tumors, most investigators agree that glial cells are the principal source (Table 17-1). A primary brain tumor is considered benign or malignant according to its behavior, but either may be lethal if it damages an especially vital part of the nervous system.

Childhood brain tumors are usually infratentorial. Adult tumors are usually supratentorial. Medulloblastomas are the most common primary brain tumors of children; gliobastomas are the most common in adults. Some rare conditions, such as tuberous sclerosis, neurofibromatosis, and von Hippel-Lindau syndrome, are associated with an increased incidence of primary intracranial tumors, but most individuals with brain tumors do not exhibit these syndromes (Table 17-2).

Much more common than primary brain tumors in adults are metastatic tumors. Breast, lung, and gastrointestinal metastases account for most of the remote cancers spreading to the central nervous system. Malignant melanoma and renal carcinoma are less common, but may be more rapidly lethal. Prostatic cancers in men may impinge on the spinal cord or the brain by extension from bony metastases. Primary spinal cord and peripheral nerve tumors account for a small fraction of all nervous system tumors.

Neuroimaging studies are essential in locating tumors, but biopsy is essential in all except those lesions that are obviously metastatic. The presence of multiple intracranial tumors with a primary malignancy outside the head suggests metastatic disease. MR and CT are both useful in identifying tumors but cannot be relied on as definitive indicators of tumor histology. Angiography is often necessary prior to surgery to establish the vascular supply to the tumor. The pattern of vessels may also suggest the type of tumor.

## PRIMARY BRAIN TUMORS

The most common primary brain tumors are the malignant (grades 3 and 4) astrocytomas. More benign astrocytomas are grades 1 and 2. Meningiomas are also common, but they occur only one third as frequently as malignant astrocytomas. Brain tumors occurring during childhood are usually neither meningiomas nor malignant astrocytomas. The more common primary brain tumors of childhood are medulloblastomas, ependymomas, and benign astrocytomas.

TABLE 17-1.  *Origin of Primary Brain Tumors*

| Category | Cell Line | Common Tumors |
|---|---|---|
| Glial | Astrocytic | Astrocytoma grade 4 (gliobastoma multiforme) |
| | | Astrocytoma grades 1 to 3 |
| | Oligodendroglial | Oligodendroglioma |
| | Ependymal | Ependymoma |
| | | Choroid plexus papilloma |
| Neural | Neuronal | Medulloblastoma |
| | Pineal | Pineoblastoma |
| Neural crest | Arachnoid | Meningioma |
| | Schwann cells | Schwannoma |
| Mesodermal | Vascular | Hemangioblastoma |
| | Pituitary | Pituitary adenoma |
| Ectodermal | Uncertain | Craniopharyngioma |

**Astrocytomas**

The location of an astrocytoma dictates treatment and prognosis as much as does its cell type. Brainstem astrocytomas are histologically often fairly benign in appearance, but they are surgically unapproachable and usually become rapidly lethal because of their location. Cerebellar astrocytomas may appear highly malignant histologically, but they are usually easily resected, and the prognosis for long-term survival of the patient is excellent. The adult grade 4 astrocytoma appears malignant histologically and is malignant behaviorally.

**Glioblastoma Multiforme.**  Astrocytoma grade 4 has traditionally been called glioblastoma multiforme. It is typically a highly malignant, rapidly lethal tumor of middle-aged adults; men being more commonly affected than women. It usually arises in the hemispheres, but may develop in the corpus callosum and extend bilaterally to form a butterfly-shaped tumor (Fig. 17-1). Signs of malignancy include variable cell types and immature astrocytes. Large multinucleated cells and numerous mitotic figures are usually evident. Hemorrhage into the tumor or necrotic foci in the tumor is common. Necrosis may be so extensive that the tumor appears to be little more than a cyst. Median survival with no treatment is 9 months from the initial appearance of symptoms. With surgical resection, chemotherapy, and radiation therapy, survival may be doubled. Regardless of treatment, 5-year survival is close to 0%.

Lower grade astrocytomas have fewer malignant features, but cell

TABLE 17-2.  *Intracranial Tumors Associated with Specific Syndromes*

| Syndrome | Tumors |
|---|---|
| Neurofibromatosis type 2 | Schwannoma, meningioma, astrocytoma, ependymoma |
| Tuberous sclerosis | Astrocytoma, ependymoma, ganglioneuroma |
| von Hippel-Lindau disease | Hemangioblastoma |
| Ataxia telangiectasia | Microglioma |
| Neurocutaneous melanosis | Leptomeningeal melanoma |

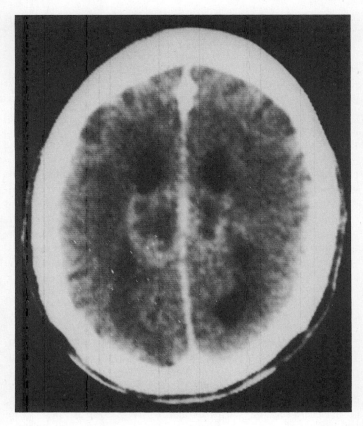

FIG. 17-1. On postcontrast CT scan, glioblastoma multiforme involving the corpus callosum may be seen crossing into both cerebral hemispheres. (From Lechtenberg, R: The Psychiatrist's Guide to Diseases of the Nervous System. New York, John Wiley and Sons, 1982.)

characteristics in one part of a tumor may appear more benign than in another part of the tumor. A malignant tumor without the high level of dedifferentiation characteristic of glioblastoma multiforme is described as a grade 3 astrocytoma. Treatment is usually unsuccessful with this tumor, but 5-year survival is about 10%.

**Astrocytoma Grades 1 and 2.**  Survival with less malignant astrocytomas is variable. With a grade 1 astrocytoma, 5-year survival may be as high as 60%. Surgery is the treatment of choice. The location of the astrocytoma is especially important in determining its lethality.

Astrocytomas originating in the cerebellum are usually benign, regardless of the histologic characteristics of the tumor. Ten-year survival of patients with cerebellar astrocytomas is better than 85%.

### Meningiomas

About 18% of primary adult intracranial tumors are meningiomas, thus making them the most common intracranial tumors of adults after glioblastoma multiforme. Because they arise from the meninges, they usually appear as a mass overlying the brain. The tumor is usually attached to the meninges by a broad base and may be associated with hyperostosis in the overlying bone. If the tumor has a narrow base, it may be mistaken for an intraparenchymal brain tumor.

Occasionally, the tumor spreads as a relatively thin sheet, a form called meningioma en plaque. Meningiomas may also arise from the tentorium cerebelli, falx cerebri, or meningeal lining of the spinal cord. Calcifications often develop in the tumors in structures called psammoma bodies. Meningiomas are generally benign in their histologic characteristics, but may be unresectable because of their location. Recurrence after resection is a major problem with this tumor type, and radiation treatment is largely ineffective. Recurrence of as many as one out of five tumors occurs even when the resection appears to be complete. Brachytherapy with implanted radioactive needles may be the only feasible treatment after multiple attempts at resection of the tumor.

### Oligodendrogliomas

Oligodendrogliomas are relatively rare, but are generally benign. They usually appear in the cerebral hemispheres, often highly superficially. Calcifications develop in more than half of them. Middle-aged adults are most commonly affected. Seizures, rather than focal deficits, are often the initial sign of tumor. The treatment of choice is surgical resection. With treatment, 5-year survival ranges from 50 to 80%.

### Ependymomas

Ependymomas affect children and adolescents five times as often as they affect adults. They usually arise in the midline of the cerebellum from the ependymal lining of the fourth ventricle, but they may develop supratentorially or below the foramen magnum. They may seed through the subarachnoid space. Resection is often attempted with inconsistent results, and radiation therapy of the craniospinal axis is usually necessary. One third to one half of the children treated for this tumor survive 10 years.

### Medulloblastomas

Medulloblastomas account for about one in four primary childhood brain tumors. They are the most common tumors of the posterior fossa in children. They usually develop in the midline of the cerebellum and produce signs and symptoms of cerebellar dysfunction or hydrocephalus. They may metastasize by spread through the CSF, but they are sensitive to radiation therapy. In fact, they are so sensitive that resection is generally unnecessary. The tumor mass and location usually produce an obstructive hydrocephalus that necessitates shunting. With shunting and radiation treatment, about one fourth to one third of the affected children survive 10 years.

## Schwannomas

Schwannomas usually develop on cranial nerve VIII, but they may develop on nerves V, IX, X, or VII in or near the cerebello-pontine angle. Bilateral schwannomas are characteristic of type 2 neurofibromatosis, a hereditary disorder associated with a defect on chromosome 11. These are fibrous, slowly growing tumors that should be removed by surgery. They characteristically produce flaring of the internal auditory canal and may be visualized readily on MR scanning with contrast enhancement. Surgical resection is often curative. These tumors are insensitive to radiation and chemotherapy. If the tumor is left untreated, the expanding mass will cause multiple cranial nerve deficits and may eventually produce lethal compression of the brainstem.

## Pinealomas

Several different tissues produce tumors in the pineal region. Most commonly, the pineal tumor contains gonadal tissue and is consequently called a germinoma or dysgerminoma. The patients usually become symptomatic during adolescence, boys being affected several times more commonly than girls. Hydrocephalus and diencephalic dysfunction may develop rapidly with tumors in this location. Surgical resection is difficult, but necessary for survival.

## Pituitary Adenomas

Pituitary adenomas invariably arise in the sella turcica and usually produce enlargement of it. Microscopic adenomas may produce symptoms long before structural changes are evident in or about the sella turcica. Extension of the tumor upward impinges on the optic chiasm and produces bitemporal hemianopia. Eosinophilic adenomas are the tumors that typically secrete growth hormone and cause gigantism in children and acromegaly in adults. Basophilic adenomas secrete ACTH and produce Cushing syndrome. Chromophobe adenomas may produce prolactin and thereby cause infertility and amenorrhea in women and impotence in men.

Although pituitary tumors may produce few symptoms for many years, they are potentially lethal or disabling and should be removed whenever possible. Hemorrhagic infarction of the pituitary tumor may produce pituitary apoplexy, a potentially lethal form of chemical meningitis and pituitary failure. Complete resection of the tumor is desirable, but with extension of the tumor into structures at the base of the brain, this may not be feasible. Transphenoidal hypophysectomy is preferred if extension above the diaphragma sellae is limited. Bromocriptine may suppress tumor growth if the adenoma is prolactin secreting, but it is not obviously superior to surgical resection. Five-year survival with surgical containment of the tumor is 80 to 95%.

## Craniopharyngiomas

These usually arise above the sella turcica in the area of the infundibulum. As they grow, they compress the pituitary inferiorly, the hypothalamus superiorly, and the optic chiasm anteriorly. They are often cystic and usually calcified. If they can be resected, the patient has an 85 to 90% chance of surviving 5 years.

## Choroid Plexus Papillomas

Tumors arising from the choroid plexus develop in both children and adults. The behavior of these tumors is variable. Prognosis is related to accessibility and histologic characteristics. Complete resection should be done whenever feasible.

## Colloid Cysts

Young adults may become symptomatic for epithelium-lined cysts in the third ventricle. These usually form in the anterior third ventricle and create symptoms, such as headache, lethargy, and nausea, when obstruction to the free flow of CSF develops. This obstruction may be acute and rapidly progressive or intermittent and exacerbated by changes in head position. Many cysts are surgically inaccessible, but shunting of CSF out of the obstructed ventricles may fully relieve the hydrocephalus and leave the patient asymptomatic.

## MANAGING HERNIATION

With many intracranial tumors, the patient is at risk of developing a herniation either transfalcially, that is, across the falx cerebri, transtentorially, that is, across the tentorium cerebelli, or transforamenally, that is, through the foramen magnum. Acute herniation in any direction may be lethal unless the displacement of brain tissue can be reversed at least partially. In intracranial tumors, this is often accomplished by administering 100 mg of dexamethasone by IV push, with 4 to 20 mg delivered by IV infusion every 4 to 6 hours. Administration of a hyperosmolar agent, such as mannitol at 2g/kg in 20% solution, is useful at the time herniation appears to be occurring. The hyperosmolar agent may transiently reduce intracerebral or intracerebellar edema and thereby slow or temporarily arrest the herniation. Continuous infusions of hyperosmolar agents are not useful.

The patient who appears to be herniating, as evidenced by deteriorating consciousness, dilating pupils, and other focal signs, should be intubated and placed on respiratory support. Hyperventilating this intubated patient helps to thwart herniation by reducing the

$P_{CO_2}$, which in turn decreases the intracranial pressure. Some physicians recommend administering a single dose of diuretic, furosemide 80 mg IV, to induce diuresis and reduce CSF formation, but the massive dose of a hyperosmolar agent, such as mannitol, usually accomplishes this diuresis and transient dehydration.

## INTRASPINAL MENINGIOMAS

Intraspinal meningiomas develop 4 times as often in women as in men. The lesions grow so slowly that symptoms, such as radicular pain and paraparesis, usually precede diagnosis by 2 to 3 years. The thoracic region is most often involved, and the lumbar region is least often involved. These tumors occasionally become embedded in the cord and appear to be intraparenchymal. Surgical removal should be attempted whenever feasible. With complete resection, the patient may have full recovery of strength and normal sensation if damage to the cord is negligible.

## METASTATIC DISEASE

About 40% of all intracranial tumors are metastatic lesions. Metastases may spread to the skull, meninges, brain, spinal cord, or subarachnoid space. Lung cancer is the most common source for metastases, with breast cancer accounting for nearly as many tumors in women. Malignant melanoma is less commonly the source than are the lungs or breast, but it is more common than tumors originating in the genitourinary tract. Leukemias, lymphomas, and gastrointestinal cancers account for about 25% of all intracranial metastases.

### Solid Tumors

Metastatic lesions in the brain usually develop at the grey-white junction. The most common symptom is headache. Cognitive impairment is the most common sign. About one fifth of patients with metastatic disease have seizures, and for half of these, seizures are the first evidence of intracranial metastases. In some patients, hemorrhage into the tumor produces acute neurologic deterioration. Malignant melanoma and choriocarcinoma are the most likely to bleed of all the metastatic lesions.

Metastatic lesions can usually be identified as neoplastic on CT or MR scanning, but that they are metastatic is only suggested by a distinctive location, such as at the grey-white junction, and by multiple foci of tumor. In some patients with cancer, the incidence of primary brain tumors is increased: breast cancer has an associated increased incidence of meningiomas. If the lesion appears to be metastatic and no primary tumor is known, then a primary locus must be sought.

In association with cancer, some patients develop nonbacterial thrombotic endocarditis, with emboli to the brain causing infarction. Those with lymphomas may develop progressive multifocal leu-

TABLE 17-3.  *Management of Intracranial Metastases*

| Tumor Type or Source | Radiosensitivity |
| --- | --- |
| Lymphoma | High |
| Seminoma | High |
| Breast | High |
| Choriocarcinoma | High |
| Lung | High to moderate |
| Esophageal | Moderate |
| Gastrointestinal | Moderate |
| Prostate | Moderate to poor |
| Melanoma | Negligible |
| Hypernephroma | Negligible |
| Sarcoma | Negligible |

koencephalopathy, a demyelinating lesion associated with immune disorders and caused by a variety of papovaviruses.

The management of metastatic disease depends on the type of tumor found (Table 17-3). Metastatic lung cancers may be sensitive to radiation therapy. High-dose steroid treatment produces at least transient improvement with a wide variety of metastatic tumors, but the cushingoid effects of the drugs limit their usefulness. Single metastases to the head from primary tumors that are not expected to be rapidly lethal should be resected if this can be accomplished without substantial injury to the patient. This generally means that the metastatic lesion must be superficial. If the tumor type is highly sensitive to radiation therapy, surgical resection may provide no advantages. The dose of radiation should be minimized to avoid the brain necrosis and dementia associated with excessive irradiation.

### Meningeal Carcinomatosis

Cancer may spread throughout the leptomeninges without producing discrete masses. This type of spread develops in about 4% of patients dying with cancer. It routinely presents with headache, dementia, radiculopathy, or cranial nerve deficits. Typically, the patient appears to have multifocal disease. Even if no cancer cells are found in the cerebrospinal fluid, the CSF is usually abnormal in terms of increased protein content, elevated white blood cell count, depressed glucose content, or elevated pressure. The results of CT or MR scanning often reveal enlarged ventricles in association with the meningeal carcinomatosis. The primary tumors most often responsible for meningeal carcinomatosis are those in the breasts, lungs, and stomach, as well as melanomas appearing in any organ. Of these, tumors in the lung and stomach are generally fairly resistant to chemotherapy and radiation when they are distributed throughout the subarachnoid space. Treatment with intrathecal administration of drugs is useful with some tumor types. Installation of an Ommaya reservoir may simplify delivery of the chemotherapy. Methotrexate is the antineoplastic drug most often delivered directly into the CSF either by lumbar puncture or by Ommaya reservoir.

## Meningeal Lymphomatosis

Intrathecal spread of lymphoma may cause signs and symptoms similar to those produced by intrathecal spread of carcinoma. This is distinct from primary brain lymphoma, a tumor that develops most commonly in patients with HIV-1 infection. The lymphoma of meningeal lymphomatosis originates outside the nervous system and metastasizes to the subarachnoid space to form sheets of cells or nodules, rather than substantial masses. Meningeal lymphomatosis is often sensitive to radiation therapy combined with chemotherapy.

## SELECTED REFERENCES

Bullard DE, Cox EB, Seigler HF: Central nervous system metastases in malignant melanoma. Neurosurgery 8:26, 1981.

Choksey MS, Valentine A, Shawdon H, et al: Computed tomography in the diagnosis of malignant brain tumors: Do all patients require biopsy? J Neurol Neurosurg Psychiatry 52: 821, 1989.

Davis JM, Zimmerman RA, Bilaniuk LT: Metastases to the central nervous system. Radiol Clin North Am 20:417, 1982.

DeAngelis LM, Delattre J-Y, Posner JB: Radiation-induced dementia in patients cured of brain metastases. Neurology 39:789, 1989.

Manz HJ: Neuropathology of systemic malignant neoplasia. Pathobiol Annu 12:233, 1982.

Wasserstrom WR, Glass JP, Posner JP: Diagnosis and treatment of leptomeningeal metastasis from solid tumors. Cancer 49:759, 1982.

*Chapter 18*
# Congenital Disorders

Birth defects affecting the nervous system usually arise from obvious developmental or infectious disorders. Intrauterine infections with a variety of viruses, such as rubella, cytomegalovirus, and HIV, routinely produce developmental disturbances that may severely impair or lethally damage the developing nervous system. Static encephalopathies that appear to have originated at or before birth are called cerebral palsy, but this broad label does not imply a single cause for all prenatal neurologic injuries. Some individuals with perinatal brain damage suffered asphyxia at the time of delivery, but many children with CNS abnormalities make poor respiratory efforts at birth and the result of the problem is confused with its cause. Many congenital neurologic problems are treatable; some produce so few deficits that treatment is unnecessary.

## CHIARI MALFORMATION

Chiari originally described four anomalies of the hindbrain; but at present, only two are considered related disturbances of hindbrain development. Type 1 involves displacement of the cerebellar tonsils into the upper cervical spinal canal, and type 2 involves caudal displacement of the medulla, pons, and vermis. Type 2 is much more complex and more likely to produce symptoms than is type 1. In type 3 of Chiari's original scheme, the cerebellum herniated into a high cervical meningocele; in type 4, a hypoplastic cerebellum was probably caused by congenital hypothyroidism. A hypoplastic cerebellum occurs with Down syndrome, as well as with cretinism and other congenital endocrine disturbances, and so is not pathognomonic for a specific disease.

The type 1 Chiari malformation is often referred to as the adult Chiari malformation because affected individuals usually become symptomatic with ataxia during the third or fourth decades of life. Type 2 is more commonly called the Arnold-Chiari malformation. Arnold described the spina bifida that is associated with some cases of the type 2 Chiari malformation.

### Type 1 Chiari Malformation

With the type 1 malformation, the cerebellar tonsils may extend a few segments down the cervical spinal canal. Hydrocephalus may develop with this condition, but syringomyelia, a cyst of the cervical spinal cord, is more likely to be the immediate cause of symptoms in the affected adult. Patients with this congenital anomaly usually manifest signs of brainstem, cervical cord, or cerebellar dysfunction over the course of months or years. The cerebellar damage may produce gait ataxia, limb clumsiness, dysarthria, and nystagmus.

146

Damage to the spinal cord from an enlarging syrinx or cyst at the cervical level usually produces a cape-like distribution of sensory change, often accompanied by insensitivity to pain in the fingers, which can allow burns and penetrating ulcers to occur. Brainstem signs include problems with swallowing, facial sensation, and balance.

Decompression of the posterior fossa is often sufficient to eliminate most symptoms. Problems referrable to a cervical or brainstem cyst will not remit with posterior fossa craniectomy.

### Type 2 Chiari Malformation

The disturbance responsible for type 2 anomalies probably occurs before the fifth week of embryonic development. The posterior fossa in the full-term infant with a type 2 anomaly is smaller than normal (Table 18-1). The tentorium cerebelli is positioned abnormally low. The caudal displacement of the cerebellar vermis may be extreme, with vermal tissue extending several segments down into the cervical spinal canal. Associated anomalies include multiple malformations of the brainstem, an enlarged interthalamic connection, a caudally displaced medulla oblongata and cervical spinal cord, and an elongated fourth ventricle. The cervicomedullary junction may be beak-shaped, and the quadrigeminal plate, which normally has two inferior and two superior colliculi, may be conical. Non-neurologic anomalies sometimes seen in association with type 2 Chiari malformation include an imperforate anus and cardiovascular malformations.

The patient with spina bifida is usually more impaired than the individual without this associated anomaly. The spinal cord in these individuals may sit much lower than is normal in the spinal canal, a position often described as tethered. With a defect in the vertebrae, spinal cord anatomy may be extremely abnormal and spinal cord functioning highly impaired. These patients are more likely than those without spina bifida to have hydrocephalus at birth or during infancy and more likely to be retarded and paraplegic.

## SYRINGOMYELIA

Syringomyelia, a cyst in the spinal cord, may occur with either Chiari malformations or the Dandy-Walker syndrome or independ-

TABLE 18-1.   *Chiari Type 2 Malformation*

| Principal Features | Common Features | Occasional Features |
| --- | --- | --- |
| Vermis caudally displaced | Hydrocephalus | Aqueductal stenosis |
| Medulla caudally displaced | Beaked cervicomedullary junction | Tentorial hypoplasia |
| Small posterior fossa | Conical tectal plate | Microgyria |
| Low tentorium cerebelli | Enlarged interthalamic bridge | Hemivertebrae |
| Atlanto-occipital fusion | Spina bifida | Klippel-Feil syndrome |
| | Syringomyelia | Foramen of Magendie cyst |

ently of either developmental disorder. The syrinx or cyst may develop at the cervical level and extend into the medulla oblongata to produce syringobulbia. Alternatively, it may develop at other levels of the cord and extend either cephalad or caudad. Some syrinxes extend the entire length of the spinal cord.

Most syrinxes extend from or connect with the central spinal canal. This central canal runs through the spinal cord gray matter. An enlarging syrinx compresses the spinal cord gray matter and produces focal or diffuse anterior horn cell disease. Damage to these motor neurons causes atrophy in the muscles controlled by the injured anterior horn cells. The anterior decussation of sensory fibers is usually disrupted by the spinal cord cyst, with focal anesthesia as the usual consequence.

Syringomyelia often develops as a congenital disorder that enlarges and produces symptoms as the patient ages. Occasionally, a glioma is responsible for the cyst formation. Attempts to halt the enlargement of the cyst and stop the damage to the cord accruing with that enlargement have involved shunts, radiation, needle punctures, and sclerosing agents, but no approach has been very successful.

## SPINA BIFIDA

Spina bifida, the failure of fusion of the dorsal elements of the vertebra, usually occurs in the lumbosacral region. It may occur in association with a Chiari malformation or independently. The bony defect is not so much a problem as is the defect in spinal cord formation that often accompanies this condition. The lining of the cord may bulge out of the defect as a meningocele, or neural, as well as leptomeningeal, elements may extend through the defect as a myelomeningocele. This is a congenital disorder that may produce paraplegia and impaired bladder and bowel control if the cord anomaly is substantial. Surgical repair of a meningocele or myelomeningocele is necessary simply to avoid recurrent meningitis, but surgical correction of the aberrant leptomeninges and neural tissue does not correct motor and sensory defects caused by the anomaly.

## DANDY-WALKER SYNDROME

The most constant features of the Dandy-Walker syndrome are a hypoplastic vermis, a cyst of the posterior fossa, enlargement of the posterior fossa and fourth ventricle, abnormally high placement of the tentorium cerebelli, and elevation of the transverse sinuses (Table 18-2). The inferior part of the cerebellum is abnormally small or undeveloped. Many other anomalies may occur in association with these congenital abnormalities. These include agenesis of the corpus callosum, inappropriately located islands of glial tissue (heterotopias), fusion of the hypothalamic nuclei, dysgenesis of the medulla oblongata, and spinal cord anomalies. Lesions outside the

TABLE 18-2.    *Dandy-Walker Malformation*

| Principal Features | Common Features | Occasional Features |
|---|---|---|
| Posterior fossa cyst | Hydrocephalus | Aqueductal stenosis |
| Dysgenesis of vermis | Agenesis of corpus callosum | Fusion of hypothalami |
| High tentorium | Neuronal and glial heterotopias | Agenesis of pyramids |
| Large posterior fossa | Agenesis of flocculi and tonsils | Syringomyelia |
| High transverse sinuses | Atresia of fourth ventricle foramina | Malformation of olives |

nervous system also appear with the Dandy-Walker malformation. These include polydactyly, spinal anomalies, cleft palate, and renal defects. Patients often exhibit hydrocephalus at birth or soon after.

The injury responsible for the Dandy-Walker malformation is presumed to occur during the sixth to seventh weeks of embryonic development. Impaired development, rather than regression of structures, appears to be the basis for the central nervous system anomalies.

Occasionally, the patient with this anomaly is asymptomatic throughout life, but more commonly, the patient has hydrocephalus. The affected child may have an enlarged head and obvious developmental delays. Hydrocephalus also may develop months or years after birth. Nausea, vomiting, lethargy, and failure to thrive may signal the development of this complication. Older children and adults who develop dysfunction with this anomaly may exhibit progressive cerebellar and cranial nerve deficits, such as gait instability and nystagmus. If hydrocephalus is responsible for the deterioration, shunting of the ventricles may be necessary. The diagnosis is usually obvious on CT or MR studies of the brain.

## CEREBRAL PALSY

Cerebral palsy includes a variety of congenital disturbances associated with static encephalopathy. The child's impairments need not be evident at birth, but the basis for impairments that subsequently appear must have been present at birth. Many of the affected individuals are presumed to have had hypoxic brain damage at or before birth, but many other prenatal and perinatal problems may produce the nonprogressive brain injuries characteristic of cerebral palsy.

Mental retardation need not be present with injuries producing cerebral palsy, but many of the affected individuals do have cognitive, affective, or seizure disorders. Evidence of cerebal palsy includes failure to achieve psychomotor milestones at the appropriate age or ever. Because this is an extremely diverse group of individuals, often with multiple impairments, no general guidelines have been formulated for treatment other than the general mandate that the child's abilities be exploited and developed as much as possible and his or her handicaps be corrected to whatever extent is feasible.

## INTRAUTERINE INFECTIONS

Intrauterine infections are a major cause of cerebral palsy. Infections that often cause brain damage circumscribed sufficiently to allow the fetus to survive include rubella, cytomegalovirus, and toxoplasmosis. Problems associated with these infections include deafness, retardation, and epilepsy.

HIV infection is readily transmitted to the fetus from an infected woman. This transmission is usually referred to as congenital AIDS, although the infant usually does not meet strict criteria for the immunodeficiency syndrome. Damage to the fetal brain includes extensive neuronal loss and perivascular calcifications. Profound retardation may be less apparent than with other intrauterine viral infections because survival for these children is usually limited to months or just a few years.

## VON HIPPEL-LINDAU SYNDROME

Patients with von Hippel-Lindau syndrome usually become symptomatic in their second or third decade of life with intracranial hemorrhages or polycystic liver disease. The major features of the syndrome include hemangioblastoma formation in the cerebellum or brainstem, retinal angiomas, and visceral cysts or tumors (Table 18-3). Besides the liver, other organs and structures that may develop cysts include the ovaries, epididymis, pancreas, and spleen. In the fourth or fifth decade of life, the affected individual is at risk for renal cell carcinoma and other renal tumors. Other types of angiomas or adenomas may develop with this syndrome, but they are less common than renal tumors.

This syndrome is inherited by autosomal dominant transmission, but penetrance is variable. Sudden death is likely if the posterior fossa hemangioblastoma is unrecognized and untreated before a massive hemorrhage occurs. Even with recognition and resection of the hemangioblastoma, the individual at risk may still die from renal cell carcinoma.

## ATAXIA TELANGIECTASIA

Of the many progressive ataxias that are transmitted in an autosomal recessive pattern, ataxia telangiectasia is one of the simplest to recognize. The child is unstable sitting and standing even after having successfully achieved these milestones. Coarse nystagmus,

TABLE 18-3.   *von Hippel-Lindau Syndrome*

| Principal Features | Common Features | Occasional Features |
|---|---|---|
| Cerebellar hemangioblastomas | Hepatic cysts | Splenic cysts |
| Retinal angiomas | Brainstem hemangioblastomas | Lung cysts |
| Renal cell carcinoma | Hepatic angiomas | Omental cysts |
| Epididymal cysts | Renal angiomas | Ovarian cysts |
| Erythrocytosis | Renal adenomas | Cerebellar cysts |
| Pheochromocytomas | Spinal hemangioblastomas | Ovarian angiomas |

trunkal tremors, and obvious clumsiness are usually evident within the first few months of life. This ataxia is associated with telangiectasias over the pinna of the ear, extending to the malar prominences and subsequently involving the conjunctivae of the eyes during the first decade of life. Dementia is evident by adolescence if not earlier and appears to be progressive. Immunoglobulin deficiencies, primarily involving IgA and IgE are also characteristic of the syndrome and may contribute to the recurrent respiratory infections that usually lead to death before the patient is 20 years old. The hereditary defect is presumed to be on chromosome 14.

## FRIEDREICH DISEASE

The most common progressive ataxia is Friedreich disease. This is transmitted in an autosomal recessive pattern, but occurs slightly more commonly in men than in women. Patients usually become symptomatic before puberty and die by the time they are 30 years old. The initial problem is usually gait difficulty. As the ataxia worsens and limb coordination deteriorates, vibration and position sense become progressively impaired, especially in the legs. Affected individuals usually develop severe dysarthria, kyphoscoliosis, and pes cavus.

Diabetes mellitus often complicates the course of this disease and the majority of patients develop hypertrophic cardiomyopathy. Neurologic damage accrues primarily in the spinal cord, rather than the cerebellum. The posterior columns and spinocerebellar tracts exhibit the most degeneration.

## VON RECKLINGHAUSEN'S NEUROFIBROMATOSIS

Neurofibromatosis occurs in several different forms. The form most likely to produce central nervous system signs and symptoms is type 2. This produces schwannomas, often bilaterally on cranial nerve VIII, and may be associated with meningiomas or gliomas. Skin lesions characteristically seen with this neurocutaneous disorder include hyperpigmented spots, called café-au-lait spots. The genetic defect giving rise to this disorder is on chromosome 22. Retardation and seizure activity are not characteristic of this disorder, but may develop if neoplasms produce cerebral damage or irritation.

Type 1 neurofibromatosis is not usually associated with acoustic schwannomas, but rather with an increased incidence of epilepsy and spinal neurofibromas. Subcutaneous neurofibromas are usually widely disseminated in patients with this disorder, and skin lesions may include axillary freckling, as well as café-au-lait spots. Optic gliomas occur less frequently with type 1 than with type 2 neurofibromatosis, but they are found in both forms of the disorder more often than would normally be expected. About 5% of patients with type 1 neurofibromatosis have CNS tumors or malignant tumors outside the CNS. Facial plexiform neurofibromas commonly disfigure individuals with type 1 neurofibromatosis.

## TUBEROUS SCLEROSIS

Tuberous sclerosis is a dominantly inherited disorder with variable penetrance. Children with this neurologic disorder may have seizures, retardation, optic gliomas, astrocytomas, and other potentially lethal neurologic complications. More severely affected individuals may exhibit adenoma sebaceum over the malar prominences of the face. Other cutaneous signs of disease include depigmented spots with serrated edges, called ash leaf spots because of their resemblance to these leaves.

## LEUKODYSTROPHY

Several hereditary demyelinating or dysmyelinating diseases produce progressive dementia, ataxia, spasticity, and sensory disturbances. The most common is metachromatic leukodystrophy, an autosomal recessive defect in aryl sulfatase A. Patients with this metabolic problem usually become symptomatic during infancy, with gait and ocular motor problems. The diagnosis usually can be made on the basis of sulfatide granules in nerve tissue as well as in tissues outside the nervous system. A peripheral nerve biopsy may establish the diagnosis. The disease progresses over the course of years and is invariably fatal.

Several types of leukodystrophy are associated with adrenal cortical degeneration. These adrenoleukodystrophies may be inherited in sex-linked recessive or autosomal dominant patterns. The patients usually become symptomatic early in life in much the same way as those with metachromatic leukodystrophy. The diseases can be distinguished by the long-chain fatty acids that accumulate in the blood in adrenoleukodystrophy. This, too, is invariably fatal, but the age of occurrence and rate of progression of the disease are variable.

Canavan disease is a leukodystrophy that is usually apparent at or soon after birth with hypotonia and macrocephaly. Intellectual development fails and optic atrophy develops in these infants. The diagnosis may be established by finding increased urinary excretion of N-acetylaspartic acid.

Pelizaeus-Merzbacher disease may have a more delayed onset than Canavan disease; progressive intellectual and motor deterioration occur over the course of years during childhood. Spasticity is a prominent feature. Autopsy studies on the brains of affected individuals reveal ferruginous deposits in the basal ganglia.

## NEURONAL CEROID LIPOFUSCINOSES

Neuronal ceroid lipofuscinosis is a common neurodegenerative disease, identified by characteristic inclusions in neuronal, as well as other, tissue. It may produce progressive dementia, ataxia, and seizures in infancy, childhood, or adult life. Affected individuals usually have associated degeneration of vision. This is a metabolic defect resulting in the accumulation of material in cells that resembles the lipofuscin routinely seen in aged neurons. The diagnosis may be made on the basis of brain biopsy, fibroblast cultures, or other tissue studies by which one can identify the characteristic intracellular inclusions. Neuroimaging studies typically reveal little more than generalized atrophy.

The metabolic defect responsible for the various types of neuronal ceroid lipofuscinosis is autosomally inherited; some families exhibit clearly autosomal dominant transmission. The enzyme defect responsible for this inborn error of metabolism is unknown.

## FRAGILE X SYNDROME

The fragile X syndrome is the most common hereditary cause of mental retardation in men. An abnormal X chromosome carries the genetic material responsible for the syndrome. This is called the fragile X syndrome because the terminal elements on the long arm of the abnormal chromosome appear stretched or broken away from the remaining elements.

Affected individuals have large ears, large testes, hypotelorism, a high, arched palate, a long, narrow face, hyperextensible joints, and prominent thumbs. Severe mental retardation is usually evident during childhood and becomes more prominent as the boy fails to achieve developmental milestones at the expected pace. Many individuals have epilepsy associated with the retardation, but the seizures are usually easily controlled with antiepileptic medication.

Women carrying the abnormal X chromosome exhibit intellectual impairment in about one third of cases, but retardation in a female carrier is much less common. No treatment affects the development of retardation in either sex. Prenatal detection of the fragile X chromosome in lymphocytes and fibroblasts allows for the detection of affected fetuses.

## SELECTED REFERENCES

Boustany R-MN, Kolodny EH: Neurological progress—the neuronal ceroid lipofuscinoses: A review. Rev Neurol *145*:105, 189.

Brown WT: The fragile X syndrome. Neurol Clin 7:107, 1989.

Gilman S, Bloedel J, Lechtenberg R: Disorders of the Cerebellum. Philadelphia, F.A. Davis, 1981.

Huson SM, Harper PS, Compston DAS: Von Recklinghausen neurofibromatosis. A clinical and population study in southeast Wales. Brain *111*:1355, 1988.

Menkes JH: The leukodystrophies. N Engl J Med *322*:54, 1989.

## Chapter 19
# Neurologic Complications of Common Medical Problems

Several medical problems have particularly destructive effects on the central and peripheral nervous system. They may cause problems indirectly, such as through a metabolic disorder that produces encephalopathy or neuropathy, or their impact may be much more direct, such as granulomatous invasion of the nervous system. Chronic alcoholism may produce hepatic encephalopathy through cumulative liver damage, but it also causes much more direct damage to the brain through Wernicke encephalopathy. Many other common medical problems also produce both direct and indirect damage to the nervous system.

## ALCOHOLISM

Alcoholism is a chronic problem that has been studied closely for many decades. Its most immediate effects on the nervous system are through nutritional disturbances and liver damage. Wernicke encephalopathy develops because of acute depletion of thiamine (vitamin $B_1$) stores in the brain. Signs of the syndrome include impaired cognitive function, such as Korsakoff (confabulatory) psychosis, disturbed ocular motor function, such as nystagmus, and gait dysfunction, such as gait ataxia. Peripheral neuropathy from chronic thiamine deficiency is often found in association with Wernicke encephalopathy, but it is not a necessary concomitant of the syndrome. Autonomic dysfunction manifested by hypothermia, orthostatic hypotension, and occasional arrhythmias develops in more severe cases of Wernicke encephalopathy and may cause death if thiamine replacement is not instituted promptly. Therapeutic doses of thiamine are 50 to 100 mg IM or IV as soon as the syndrome is recognized. The thiamine dose is usually repeated daily for 3 to 5 days after the initial dose to help rebuild thiamine stores. Wernicke encephalopathy is most often precipitated by an infusion of glucose or oral glucose load given to a chronically thiamine-depleted alcoholic individual.

Other causes of disturbed cognition with alcoholism include hepatic encephalopathy with progressive cirrhosis and acute intoxication with alcohol. Alcohol intoxication is easily diagnosed, but differentiating a hepatic encephalopathy from Wernicke encephalopathy may be more difficult when either is severe.

Individuals experiencing alcohol withdrawal face two common problems, seizures and delirium tremens. Alcohol is an effective antiepileptic, so patients usually do not have seizures while their serum alcohol levels are rising; but alcohol, like barbiturates, increases the risk of seizure activity as its serum level falls. The type of seizure exhibited depends on focal abnormalities in the patient's brain. Either generalized or partial seizures may occur with alcohol withdrawal, but the patient with no antecedent head trauma or strokes usually has a generalized tonic-clonic seizure.

Delirium tremens is an acute cognitive disorder associated with visual or auditory hallucinations, agitation, paranoia, and limb tremors. This develops in some chronically alcoholic individuals when the serum alcohol content drops to negligible levels. It is usually managed by administration of high-dose benzodiazepine such as chlordiazepoxide at 50 mg 4 to 6 times daily, although the efficacy and wisdom of this approach are still somewhat controversial. Benzodiazepine abuse among alcoholics is a major problem in some countries, so substantial reasons exist to use less abused substances, such as phenobarbital, to suppress the delirium tremens.

Some individuals with chronic alcoholism develop rapidly progressive demyelination of the corpus callosum as part of the Marchiafava-Bignami syndrome. The neurologic signs and symptoms associated with this fulminant demyelination are not specific for this syndrome; patients usually have a rapid deterioration of consciousness as focal motor and sensory deficits evolve. Autopsy examination of the brain usually has been necessary to establish the diagnosis.

Even without other signs of obvious brain damage, the chronically alcoholic patient usually develops cerebellar atrophy (Fig. 19-1). The superior vermis is the part of the brain most consistently atrophied with chronic alcohol abuse. Because many of the signs of acute alcohol intoxication, including ataxia and dysarthria, are signs of cerebellar dysfunction, the cerebellum must be considered especially vulnerable to transient and permanent effects of ethanol.

Myopathy also develops as an acute or chronic problem. Polymyositis from alcohol abuse usually produces proximal limb weak-

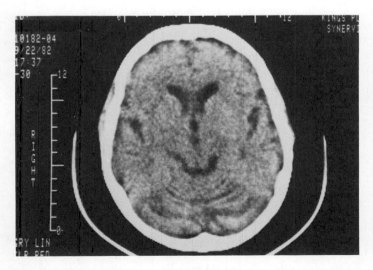

FIG. 19-1. The folia of the cerebellum are evident as ripples in the lower half of this CT scan. Cerebellar atrophy is pronounced in this patient and may have been related to chronic alcoholism.

ness associated with creatine kinase elevation in the serum. In many individuals, the extent of muscle damage is related to the total dose of alcohol ingested over the course of years.

## COCAINE ABUSE

Cocaine abuse has appeared episodically in industrialized countries over the past century. Cocaine has proven to be highly addictive, regardless of the route of administration. Its principal neurologic effects are the induction of hyperactivity, agitation, paranoia, and seizures. Cardiac arrhythmias also occur with cocaine ingestion, perhaps in part as an autonomic dysfunction induced by the drug. It is this cardiac problem, rather than the neurologic problems, that may be lethal.

Seizures occur with cocaine ingestion rather than withdrawal. The route used to acquire the drug and the dose of drug administered are less relevant to whether seizures develop than is the individual's susceptibility to seizure activity. People with epilepsy are obviously at high risk of seizure activity with cocaine use. The seizure activity and psychiatric effects of the drug are usually transient, but injuries sustained during cocaine-induced seizures may be disabling or fatal. Addiction to cocaine is somewhat atypical in that the individual need not feel a daily craving for the drug to be authentically addicted.

## OPIATE ABUSE

Most of the neurologic damage associated with opiate abuse is indirect. Heroin abusers may develop seizures with administration of the drug, but in many cases, the basis for the seizure may be other substances, such as amphetamines, phencyclidine, or cocaine, adulterating the heroin. Intravenous heroin users often develop valvular heart disease because they do not use sterile technique during self-injection. This valvular disease may help initiate subacute or acute bacterial endocarditis. This, in turn, produces mycotic aneurysms that can result in subarachnoid hemorrhages or brain abscesses with attendant intracranial-mass effects. The recent proliferation of AIDS in the intravenous-drug abusing population complicates the evaluation of these individuals. Neurologic signs and symptoms in opiate abusers may be complications of HIV encephalopathy, toxoplasma granulomas, primary central nervous system lymphomas, or other problems commonly seen in HIV-infected individuals.

## DIABETES MELLITUS

In patients with diabetes mellitus, the peripheral nervous system and the eyes are especially vulnerable to injury. Problems in the peripheral nerves are of several types, the most common being symmetric sensory neuropathy, mononeuritis multiplex, diabetic

TABLE 19-1.   *Neurologic Effects of Hypoglycemia*

| Symptoms | Signs |
|---|---|
| Headache | Disorientation |
| Generalized weakness | Tremor |
| Nausea | Vomiting |
| Visual obscuration | Seizures |
| Lethargy | Coma |

amyotrophy, and dysautonomia. Sensory neuropathy usually affects the feet earlier than it affects the hands and follows a glove-and-stocking pattern of distribution. Paresthesias are common but not usually painful. Loss of sensation and poor superficial perfusion increase the risk of perforating skin ulcers. The mononeuritis multiplex pattern affects major nerves with both sensory and motor components. It usually produces transient loss of nerve function, with recovery more typically than not occurring over the course of months. Diabetic amyotrophy and mononeuritis multiplex probably both result from specific types of vascular injuries. With diabetic amyotrophy, the patient usually develops limb girdle weakness associated with some proximal limb pain. This weakness may resolve over the course of weeks or months. Neither the symmetric sensory neuropathy nor the dysautonomia associated with diabetes mellitus remit spontaneously, and often both are resistant to improved control of the diabetes. With dysautonomia, men have impotence and both men and women have postural hypotension, as well as bladder and bowel dysfunction.

Diabetic damage to the eye is largely vascular. Proliferative retinopathy and central retinal artery occlusion may both occur and produce progressive or sudden loss of vision. Microaneurysms forming on the retina often bleed. Laser treatment of the retina may save central vision in patients with diabetes by reducing the neovascularity that extends onto the fovea and obscures macular vision.

Managing diabetes mellitus has its own risks. Hypoglycemia from insulin excess produces many transient neurologic signs and symptoms, including headache, confusion, seizures, and coma (Table 19-1). Some patients develop focal neurologic deficits, such as hemiplegia, aphasia, or cortical blindness. These deficits are transient but are not merely postictal.

## UREMIA

The neurologic complications of uremia are myriad and range from uremic encephalopathy to peripheral neuropathy. Seizures, dementia, mononeuritis multiplex, progressive sensory neuropathies, and other chronic and acute neurologic problems develop in patients with renal insufficiency. Additional problems faced by patients since the introduction of renal dialysis include a variety of dysequilibrium syndromes, such as headache or seizures associated with abrupt electrolyte changes, and dialysate-associated neuropathies.

# PREGNANCY

Central and peripheral nervous system problems may develop during pregnancy. Some, like carpal tunnel syndrome and pseudotumor cerebri, usually require no treatment, whereas others, such as seizures and strokes, usually require immediate and continuing attention.

With pregnancy, women may develop seizure disorders that were not evident before, or they may exhibit increased intracranial pressure (pseudotumor cerebri) that resolves completely with termination of the pregnancy. If seizures are associated with hypertension and proteinuria, the woman is presumed to have toxemia of pregnancy, or eclampsia. Obstetricians have traditionally used magnesium sulfate to manage the seizures associated with eclampsia, but this is inappropriate. Antiepileptic medications such as carbamazepine or phenytoin should be used to manage seizures that cannot be suppressed by correcting any apparent electrolyte abnormalities. Women with epilepsy who become pregnant have traditionally been treated with phenobarbital, but this too is inadvisable since the incidence of birth defects in women who take phenobarbital during their pregnancies is two to three times greater than that observed with phenytoin, carbamazepine, or divalproex sodium. The drug with the lowest incidence of well-documented birth defects associated with its use is carbamazepine. If an antiepileptic agent can be chosen for use during pregnancy before pregnancy occurs, it should be carbamazepine. The dose of antiepileptic medication must be monitored carefully during pregnancy because the levels of most antiepileptics are affected by the stage of the pregnancy. Drug breakdown usually accelerates as the pregnancy progresses.

During delivery, neurologic catastrophes may occur, but rarely do. These catastrophes include pituitary necrosis and subarachnoid hemorrhages. Seizures may occur during delivery or shortly thereafter because of the trauma of the event or because of idiosyncratic reactions to anesthetic and analgesic agents. Any patient developing seizures while straining during delivery must be investigated for subarachnoid hemorrhage. A CT of the head may suffice to reveal the blood. An angiogram is appropriate in cases of apparent bleeding.

Strokes occur with greater frequency during pregnancy than between pregnancies, with venous or sinous thromboses accounting for many of these cerebrovascular accidents. These are often ischemic infarctions, but hemorrhages may occur with unsuspected vascular malformations or aneurysms. If the woman has a congenital vascular malformation, the risk of bleeding from this malformation increases during pregnancy and delivery. Premature termination of the pregnancy may be necessary in this situation to avoid life-threatening complications for the mother.

Myasthenia gravis may evolve or appear during pregnancy. The children of myasthenic mothers are often born with neonatal myasthenia, a transient weakness attributable to acetylcholine receptor antibodies. The weakness may persist for months or years.

## SELECTED REFERENCES

Allredge BK, Lowenstein DH, Simon RP: Seizures associated with recreational drug abuse. Neurology *39:*1037, 1989.

Bag S, Behari M, Ahuja GK, Marmarkar MG: Pregnancy and epilepsy. J Neurol *236:*311, 1989.

Baron R, Heuser K, Marioth G: Marchiafava-Bignami disease with recovery diagnosed by CT and MRI: Demyelination affects several CNS structures. J Neurol *236:*364, 1989.

Brown WA (ed): Endocrinology of Neuropsychiatric Disorders. Neurologic Clin *6:*1, 1988.

Choy-Kwong M, Lipton RB: Seizures in hospitalized cocaine users. Neurology *39:*425, 1989.

Duncan R, Hadley D, Bone I, et al: Blindness in eclampsia: CT and MR imaging. J Neurol Neurosurg Psychiatry *52:*899, 1989.

Eymard B, Morel E, Dulac O, et al: Myasthenia and pregnancy: Clinical and immunologic study of 42 cases. Rev Neurol *145:*696, 1989.

Lechtenberg R, Sher J: AIDS in the Nervous System. New York, Churchill-Livingstone, 1989.

Lindboe CF, Loberg EM: The frequency of brain lesions in alcoholics: Comparison between 5-year periods 1975–1979 and 1983–1987. J Neurol Sci *88:*107, 1988.

Mas JL, Guegen B, Bouche P, et al: Chorea and polycythaemia. J Neurol *232:*169, 1985.

Mooradian AD: Diabetic complications of the central nervous system. Endocr Rev *9:*346, 1988.

Riggs JE (ed): Neurologic manifestations of systemic disease. Neurol Clin *7:*447, 1989.

Urbano-Marquez A, Estruch R, Navarro-Lopez F, et al: The effects of alcoholism on skeletal and cardiac muscle. N Engl J Med *320:*409, 1989.

# Index

Note: Page numbers in *italics* indicate figures; those followed by *t* indicate tables.